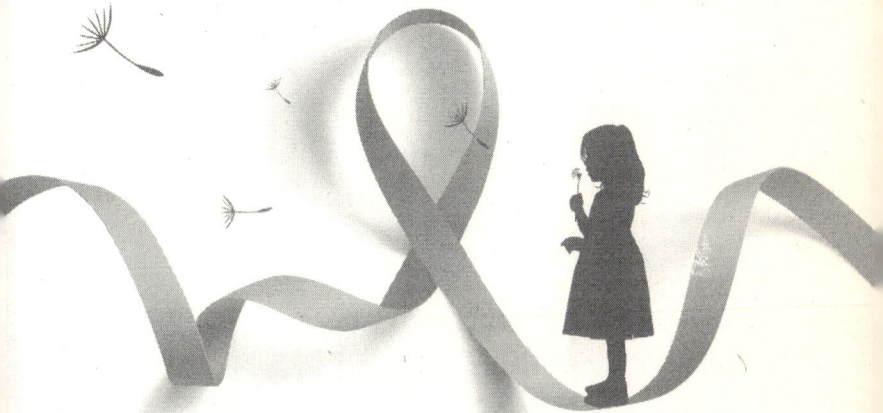

STEPHEN BENNETT

In Her Best Interests

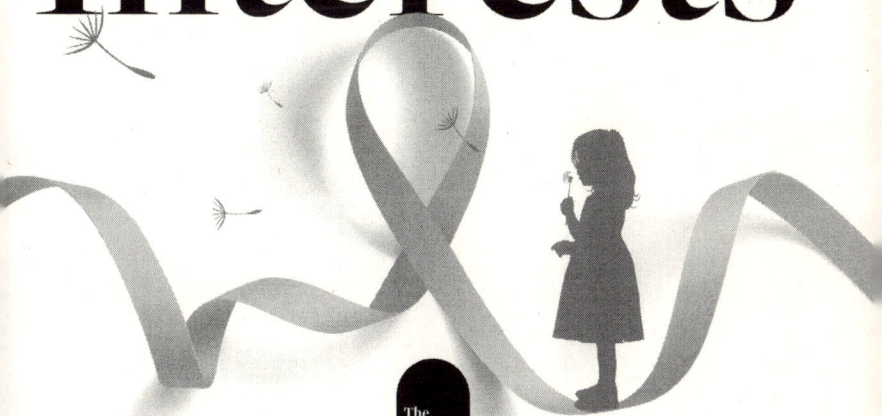

The
Book
Guild

First published in Great Britain in 2025 by
The Book Guild Ltd
Unit E2 Airfield Business Park,
Harrison Road, Market Harborough,
Leicestershire. LE16 7UL
Tel: 0116 2792299
www.bookguild.co.uk
Email: info@bookguild.co.uk
X: @bookguild

The manufacturer's authorised representative in the EU
for product safety is Authorised Rep Compliance Ltd,
71 Lower Baggot Street, Dublin D02 P593 Ireland (www.arccompliance.com)

Typeset in 11pt Minion Pro

Printed and bound in Great Britain by CMP UK

ISBN 978 1835742 129

British Library Cataloguing in Publication Data.
A catalogue record for this book is available from the British Library.

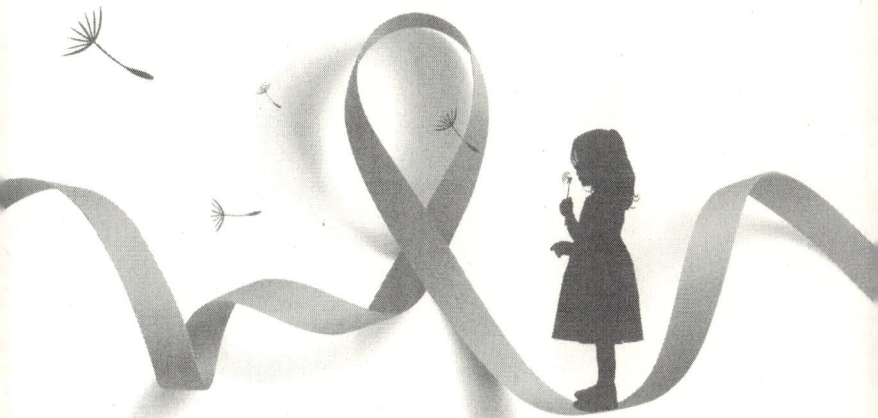

~ For each of the 400,000 childhood cancer warriors
diagnosed worldwide every year and their families ~

Even one is too many

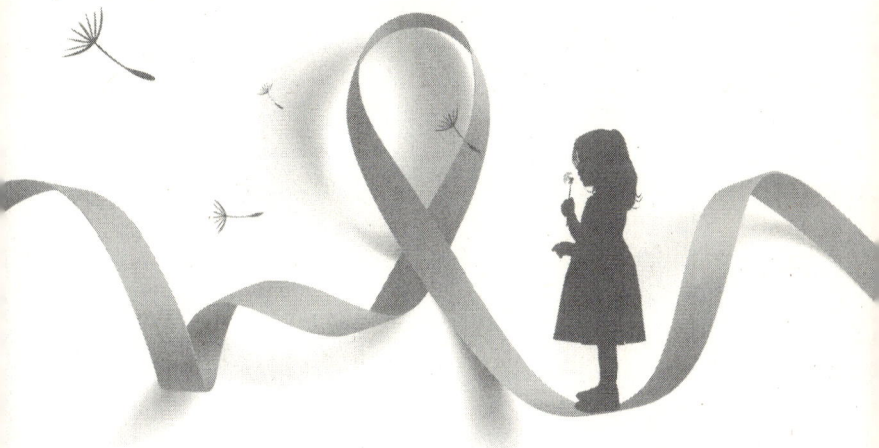

Contents

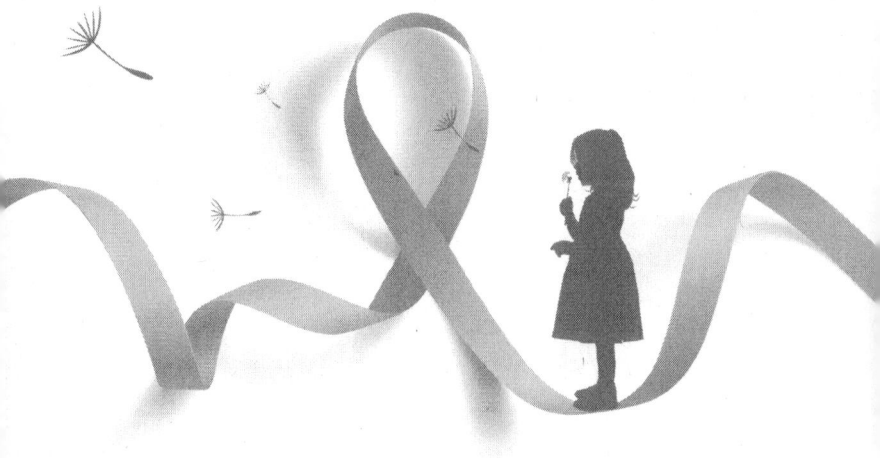

Acknowledgements

Claire, Phoebe and Leah – my world plus one.

Ms Jo Minford – our fairy godmother.

The Prof. – for never giving up.

The rest of the surgical magicians at Alder Hey – for your personal and professional bravery.

The team on Ward 3B at Alder Hey – the greatest team in the greatest children's hospital in the world.

The hundreds of other staff at Alder Hey Children's Hospital and the Clatterbridge Cancer Centre – for making Leah feel like the only child in the place every time she visited.

The many charities that supported us and so many other families on one of life's toughest journeys.

Our two incredible families, who picked us up from the floor every time we stumbled.

Everyone that picked our family members up from the

floor every time they stumbled.

Mike – for all your help, support and advice.

Marie – for your strength, love and light. We miss you every day.

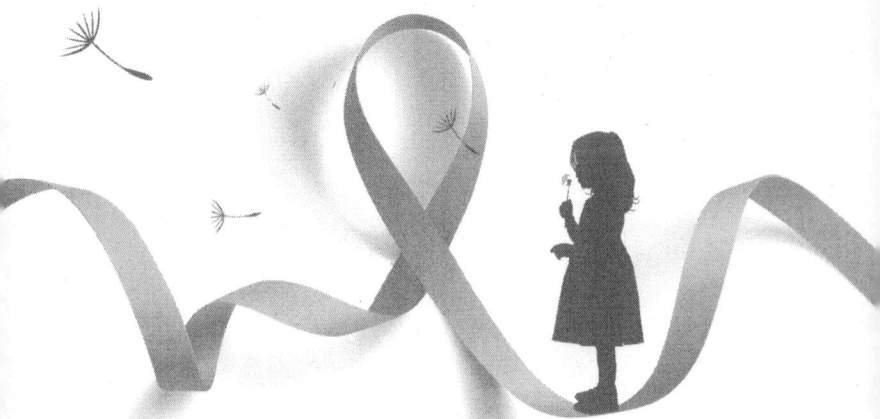

Hope is being able to see that there is light despite all of the darkness.

Desmond Tutu

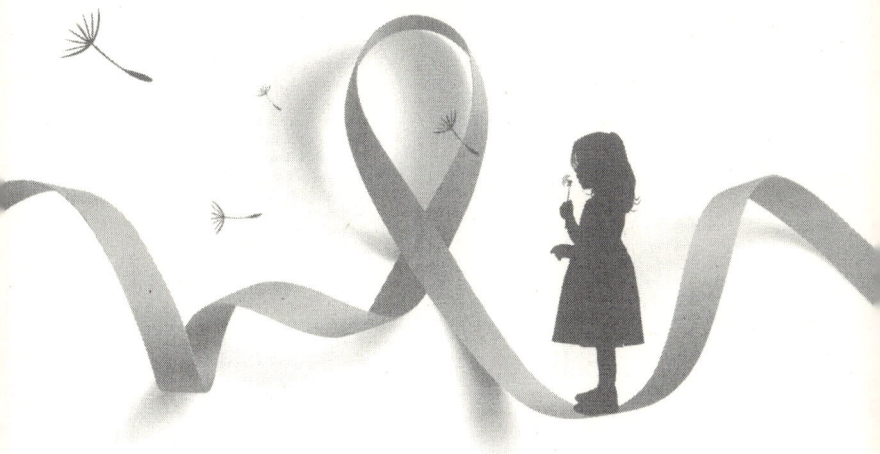

Introduction

Every so often, for some people, a moment happens. A seismic moment. One that changes everything. In a heartbeat. That moment can be planned or it can be unplanned. It can change your life for better. It can change your life for worse.

One thing, though, is certain. Once the moment has been and gone, there is nothing we can do to change it. It is already in the past. The challenge it leaves us with as individuals is how we react or respond to it. It is this response that will ultimately determine the lasting impact of the moment on the rest of our lives and potentially on the lives of those around us.

This book describes the events before and after one of those moments for me. A moment that, in turn, created life-changing moments for many other people. It is a story of tragedy, of love, of courage, of despair, of joy and, most of all, it is a story of hope (and magpies).

The life events described in this book are deeply personal and (still) deeply painful for me and for many others in my close family. This is a personal account of events in my life and all opinions and views portrayed are my own. I have altered the names of some of the people in this book to protect them. However, this is a story that I feel compelled to tell in the hope that it perhaps reaches just one person or one family, for whom it may bring a flicker of light that they so desperately need.

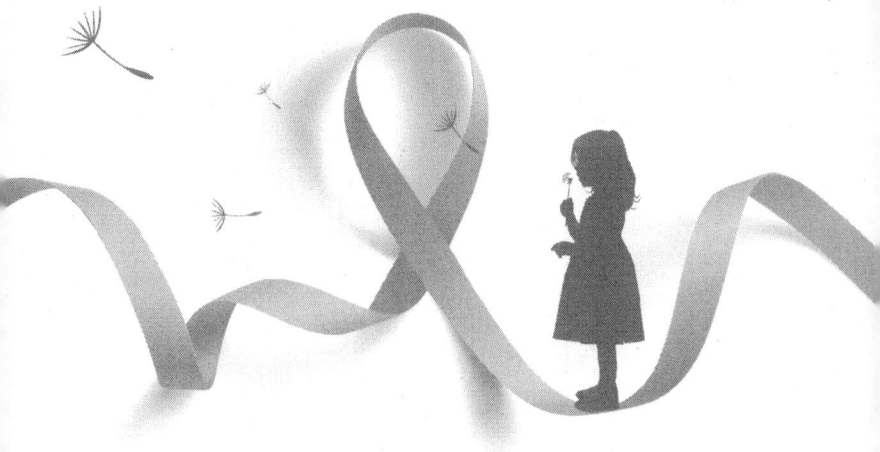

Four Words

'There is really no easy way to say this, Mr and Mrs Bennett... we think... your child has cancer.'

Four words. Four simple words.

Your

Child

Has

Cancer.

These words can never be unheard. They can never be misunderstood. They are words that you think are only ever spoken to people you see in television soaps or drama series. They can never be said to you. No, no. Your child is healthy, after all... right?

These words stop time momentarily. They also change your whole life forever in an instant. They create a moment that becomes indelibly etched into your memory. A permanent scar. Something that is ugly and painful and you dearly wish to erase or remove, but you know you probably never will.

I will never forget the very moment they were uttered to me. Where I was. Who was with me in that room. What I was wearing. The tidal wave of emotions that immediately followed them... confusion, anger, frustration, denial, despair and even a pang of guilt. Emotions that burst out of my body so violently, it left me without the energy to stand up.

I only have a handful of these powerful moments from the whole of my forty-four years on this planet. They all sit permanently and vividly inside my head. Two of the others are the moments when my girls were born. Day-to-day, I generally struggle to remember my own bloody phone number or the date, but I remember the exact time my girls were born, what they weighed, where I was stood, what colour the walls were. Moments of pure, natural beauty imprinted forever inside my mind.

These four simple words now threaten to overshadow all those other moments. They threaten to take them all away and I don't think I can do anything about it.

I'm not sure anyone else can either.

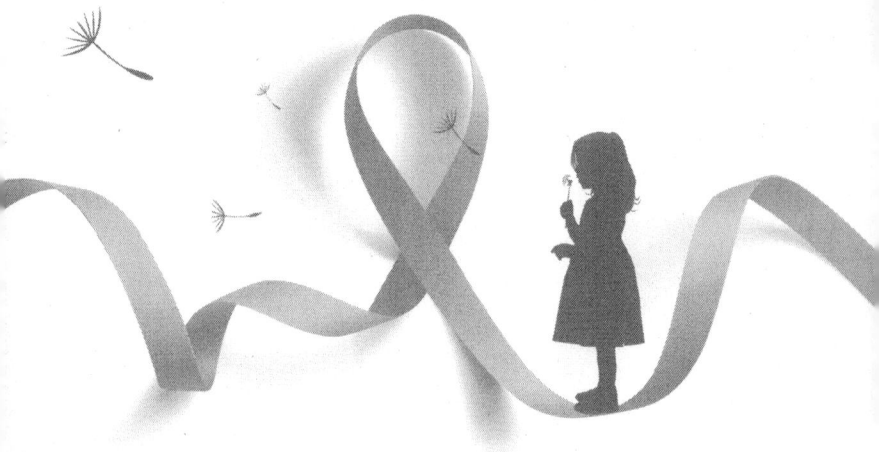

Bella and the Superglue

Saturday 17th December 2016

I'm upstairs in my youngest daughter Leah's bedroom, putting some freshly ironed clothes away in her wardrobe. I turn around quickly and bump into the chest of drawers at the side of her bed. Her bedside lamp wobbles and falls onto her bed. At the same time, a small pink fairy ornament that stood on the other end of the chest of drawers wobbles and falls onto the floor.

The bedside lamp is thankfully okay. I say thankfully because my wife, Claire, will absolutely murder me if I've broken it. I don't think she's paid it off yet on her bloody Next account. The small fairy ornament, however, is less fortunate.

The ornament has been given the name 'Bella' by Leah. Bella's a cute little thing. She was given to Leah by someone in our family when she was a baby. She has stood proudly holding her wand and displaying her fairy wings next to Leah's bed every day since. It's more or less the week before Christmas and clumsy Dad has gone and knocked her over. She now lies on Leah's bedroom carpet. Her head is staring up at me, still smiling despite now being decapitated from her body. It is like some kind of *Toy Story*/snuff movie mash-up. Bella's magic wand with a little star on the top has broken out of her hand, too, and lies about two feet away.

I scoop up the various pieces from around the room and carry her downstairs for a short session with a tube of superglue. I know if I'm quick, Leah will never notice (#DadSkills).

Wednesday 5th April 2017

I drive into work this morning feeling great. It is one of those beautiful, crisp spring mornings. The sun is shining and it is too early in the year for my hay fever to ruin it all.

I've been in my new job at Warrington Hospital for almost five months now and I'm really enjoying it. Family life is great; the girls are both settled and doing well at school. Things are pretty damn good. Every traffic light I hit seems to be green this morning, too. Then, the icing on my big fat smug cake arrives when my all-time favourite Oasis song comes on the radio. I belt out 'She's Electric' at full volume with my windows down as I make my way towards the hospital site. It is a poor man's 'Carpool Karaoke', if I'm honest, but I couldn't care less.

The morning at work passes without anything eventful happening. A couple of typical NHS meetings that add very little value, followed by an hour reading through the latest national guidance around operational planning. Just after lunch, my mobile phone buzzes and I pull it out of my pocket. Claire's name is on the screen.

Claire's mum, Marie, had been for a hospital appointment recently after being referred due to concerns about recent kidney pain and traces of blood in her urine. Claire is understandably a little anxious about the appointment. My own mum had been in hospital a few months earlier with kidney stones after having had the same symptoms, so we are just waiting on news of the confirmation of a similar diagnosis. I answer the call.

'Ste,' says Claire. Just from the tone of her voice, I can immediately tell that something is wrong. 'It's my mum.' She pauses. 'They think she has cancer.' Her voice is wobbly and I can hear she is in tears on the other end of the phone.

'Oh no, honey, I'm so sorry,' I respond. What a lame response it is, but what else do you say in a moment like that? 'Are you at home?' I ask her.

'Yes,' she replies, her voice still quivering.

'I'm on my way.'

I arrive home about thirty minutes later. I walk through the front door and Claire is stood there in tears, looking heartbroken. I throw my arms around her and we stand together in the hallway for about five minutes. Nobody saw this news coming.

Tuesday 9th May 2017

Marie went into hospital today to have her right kidney removed. The last few weeks have been a bit of a whirlwind after she was diagnosed. Claire and her family have been amazing, really. After the initial shock of the diagnosis, the whole family (led by Marie herself) have been really positive over recent weeks and have rallied around each other. It's been incredible to see the family unit kick in and create a force stronger than any degree of fear that any of them may hold individually.

Marie's operation has apparently gone well and she should be back home in a couple of days. The early indication from the surgeon suggests that they believe they have removed all the cancer with the removal of the kidney. That is all anyone could hope for at this stage and hearing that news has been a huge relief for everyone.

Thursday 8th June 2017

A month on from the procedure and Marie seems to have recovered incredibly well physically. She's been told that the team at the hospital believe there is no longer evidence of any disease, which is fantastic news. Mentally, though, Marie appears to be struggling to come to terms with what has happened. None of us, including her, saw all this coming.

It has been a matter of months since she retired from work with grand plans to travel the world with her husband, Peter (Claire's dad). The thought of having to deal with a cancer battle was nowhere on the radar and it has really affected Marie psychologically. Ever since I have known her, she has been such a strong and positive woman, and the events of the last couple of months appear to have really hurt her. She seems a lot quieter and more subdued than usual when I speak to her and she's angry about what's happened. I guess this is probably not an uncommon reaction to something so challenging.

I can't pretend to understand how difficult this must be for her, but I only hope that, in time, she will find a way to put this behind her and find her happiness again, because it is just awful seeing her so mentally tortured.

Monday 16th October 2017

Marie has been to see her consultant today at the Clatterbridge Cancer Centre over on the Wirral. Every time she has been back to see him, the sense of anxiety within Claire's whole family is palpable. I hadn't had a call from Claire during worktime, so I assumed no news was good news.

I arrive home from work in the evening and ask Claire if she knows how her mum got on. Claire has been in work today, too, and hasn't heard anything from either her mum or her dad all day. She doesn't say anything specifically, but I can tell she hasn't taken the 'no news to be good news' in the same way I have. She's only been home from work for around twenty minutes when she decides to go round to her mum and dad's to speak to them herself. She calls me around an hour later.

Marie has been told that they removed her kidney too

late and the cancer has already spread beyond the location of her surgery. It is now visible in her liver. No news is, in fact, devastating news.

Wednesday 29th November 2017

Among all the darkness that seems to have surrounded our family over recent weeks and months, today there was finally something much more positive to talk about. My younger sister, Sarah, and her partner, Phil, announced that they are now engaged. Phoebe and Leah are absolutely over the moon to find out that she has asked them to be her bridesmaids. The excitement is tinged with a tiny amount of disappointment, though, as they'll have to wait until 2019 for the big day.

Saturday 14th April 2018

A few weeks ago, my aunt tagged me in a post on Facebook from a local football team advertising that they were starting up a new girl's football team. She thought that it might be something one of the girls would be interested in. I asked them both if they fancied giving it a go. Phoebe immediately shot me the 'Are you really asking me that question, Dad?' look. That will be a no from her. Leah, on the other hand, immediately said yes.

Today, I'm taking her along to the first session. She is a little nervous at first joining in with the other girls, some of whom are a good few years older than her. She is one of the youngest in the group and comfortably the smallest, but, by the end of the session, she seems to be enjoying herself. On the way home, she is buzzing about it and can't wait to tell Claire when we get back to the house.

Having two girls, I wasn't really holding out much hope of becoming a 'Footy Dad', but maybe, just maybe, I might get the chance after all!

Tuesday 3rd July 2018

Leah is a pain in the arse getting out of bed this morning. She's really tired and doesn't want to get up for school at all. After shouting up to her about twenty-five times, I eventually have no choice but to stamp up the stairs to her room to bellow at her to get out of bed and get ready for school. When I say stamp, I *mean* stamp. They have to know, without a shadow of a doubt, you're coming up to them. I find the stamp is a great way to build up that sense of anxiety that may just spark them into corrective action. It's all about the theatre (#MoreDadSkills).

I reach her room and she dives out of bed as soon as my hand touches the door handle. I burst into the room and she looks at me as if to say, 'See, Dad, I told you I was out of bed.'

'*Get ready for school!*' I yell at her and then turn and slam her door behind me.

'Well done, Dad!' I hear her say from the other side of the door. In slamming it, I've shaken her Bella statue on her bedside table and it is now lying on her carpet 'de-wanded' again. That's another date for me with the superglue this evening… FFS!

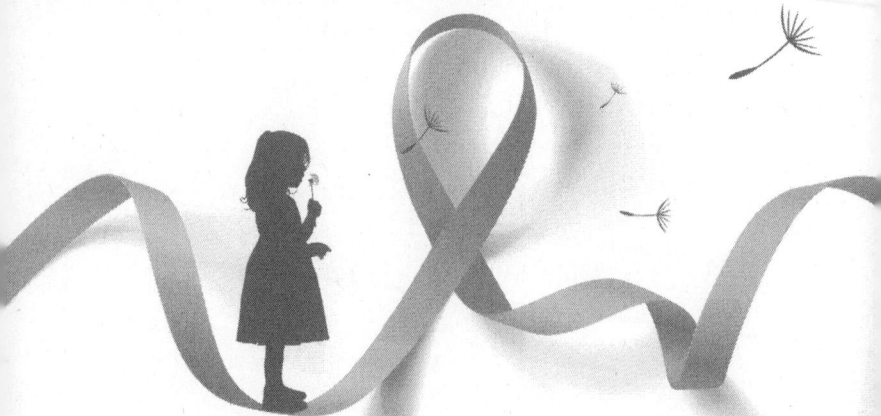

Those Annoying People

Everyone knows one of those annoying people to whom life seems to come easy. They appear to breeze through effortlessly. If you don't know someone like that, then it's probably you. While I certainly didn't realise it at the time, that was definitely me... I was that annoying person.

I have enjoyed a good career to date and I've always loved what I do. My first job out of university was in the management accounts team at Aintree University Hospital in Liverpool. I left the NHS for a short period to work in the finance team of a private sector manufacturing firm before returning twelve months later. I really missed the diversity of working in the health service. More than anything, though, I missed the people. NHS people are just the best in the world. I only realised that once I'd left.

I stayed at Aintree for around eight years in total, working my way slowly through the finance ranks. Along the way, I picked up my accountancy qualifications and now I was ready to really challenge the order! After a short period working at the main hospital in Bolton, I ended up in a finance manager's role at Alder Hey Children's Hospital in Liverpool.

During my time there, I met so many incredible people. People who were totally committed and passionate about their jobs. It's difficult to explain but I can honestly say that I've never worked in a place where I have felt part of something so special. Everyone that worked there seemed to love what they do. I imagine a good few would probably work there for free if they needed to, as they loved the place so much. It might be because it's a children's hospital and I think you have to be a bit like that to work in those places.

And so, it was with a heavy heart I walked out of Alder Hey for the last time on Thursday 10th December 2016. I felt genuinely sad getting into my car and driving out of the car park for the final time – although I knew I wouldn't miss the bloody temperamental car park barriers that seemed determined to wind me up at least once a week. I swear Ant and Dec must have been controlling them from some TV studio somewhere.

From Alder Hey, my career journey took me away from the world of finance and, yet again, away from Liverpool. On Monday 14th November 2016, I started my new job at Warrington and Halton Teaching Hospitals NHS Foundation Trust. The NHS loves a ridiculously long title.

I remember feeling nervous and excited in equal measure when I started. I was stepping into a brand-new role heading up the Transformation (service improvement) team after fourteen years working in NHS finance. I genuinely love the NHS and I'm passionate about protecting it. I've always wanted to do my bit to make it the best it can be. Therefore, the chance to lead a team of equally enthusiastic individuals to do just that felt like the only thing that could prise me away from Alder Hey.

Life was going pretty damn well for me, I have to say. Outside work, I had a fabulous family. I married an incredible woman called Claire and we had two beautiful daughters called Phoebe and Leah. We lived in a lovely home in an amazing community. Generally, I considered myself to be very lucky (I did warn you I was annoying!). In a heartbeat, though, life can change.

Sometimes it changes for the better, but sometimes it unfortunately changes for the worse. In my case, it was most definitely the latter. It really doesn't matter who you are, where you come from or how comfortable your life has been, it can all change in a split second.

From the moment I heard those 'four words', my previously perfect life disappeared. The universe had decided to throw a few hand grenades at us and run away. All of sudden, there was a seemingly infinite path of questions and challenges, anxiety and uncertainty before me. It had taken the place of my stable and happy life and I felt completely lost.

I don't really know whether the stability I had in my life was a help or a hindrance in terms of preparing me for what was to come. I had never really experienced anything I would describe as real trauma during my childhood or early adulthood. This probably meant I was hideously under-skilled and under-equipped for what lay ahead. The stability, love and strength of my family unit had probably protected me from experiencing earlier traumatic experiences. However, those things also meant that I had some serious emotional assets to draw upon when things got tough.

As a result of what has happened since the moment of hearing those four words, I now have a very different perspective on life. Even now though, despite everything... I do still consider myself to be lucky.

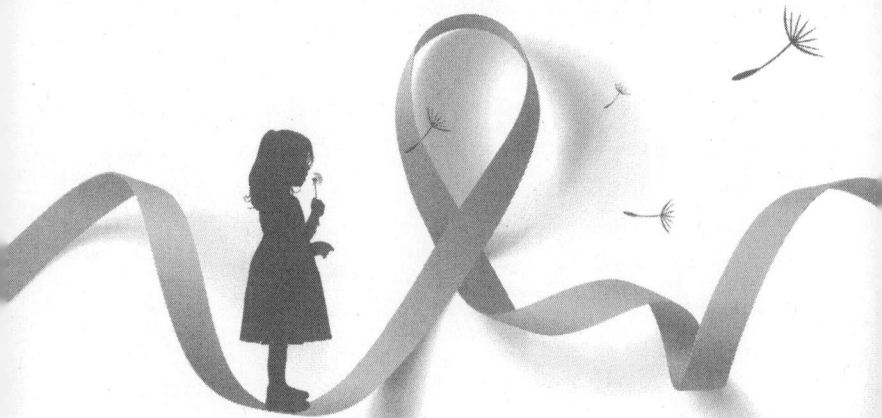

Plus One

Leah turned six on the 22nd of August. Unfortunately for her, as her birthday falls in the school summer holidays, many of her friends are usually away on holiday. Therefore, we arranged her birthday party for today. She randomly asked for a circus-themed party this year, so, over the last few weeks, we've all been busy making hook-a-duck stalls, a coconut shy, a big top scene and an area with juggling balls and a diabolo. We've also hired a face-painter and a kid's entertainer to keep her and all her school friends busy.

At the party, we have the usual rounds of pass the parcel and I've been given the high-pressure job of stopping the music at intervals. I watch covertly to make sure that different kids get to peel off the layers. Every one of the boys hangs onto the parcel for dear life when it reaches them, before eventually handing it over with a vice-like grip to the child next to them. I make sure the music doesn't stop on them. I possibly enjoy the power that comes with the role a little too much.

Halfway through the afternoon, Leah walks over to the entertainer and whispers something into her ear. Two minutes later, she is stood on the little stage with a microphone in her hand singing, 'A Million Dreams' from the film *The Greatest Showman* in front of everyone. I get a little emotional listening to her. I just love her confidence and the fact that she's completely taken the liberty to do whatever she wants given that it's her party. Regardless of whether her guests wanted to hear it, they are getting a song. I imagine that's how Jane McDonald started.

Friday 21st September 2018

Today is Marie's birthday, so we're all going round to Claire's parents' house for a takeaway this evening. When we arrive, I notice Marie looks pale, but she seems happy to see the family together to celebrate with her. She's recently been put on new chemotherapy medication to help control her condition as much as possible, but the side effects of the drugs have not been insignificant. She's been really up and down physically. Her feet have been blistering and sore, meaning she's struggled to walk on occasion. She has also lost much of her appetite, meaning she has visibly started to lose a bit of weight. I notice she doesn't really eat much of her chicken korma tonight.

Despite all the challenges she faces, though, she always makes the effort to ensure everyone is comfortable and enjoying themselves. It's really quite inspiring but heartbreaking in equal measure.

Tuesday 13th November 2018

It has been another fairly mundane day at work. Back-to-back meetings talking about tasks that haven't been completed. The irony is that the tasks probably could have been completed if we weren't all sat in back-to-back meetings all day discussing them.

I arrive back home at around six o'clock in the evening. I come in and the girls are both sat in the front room watching TV. Phoebe jumps up and gives me a big hug and then Leah does the same. Regardless of how dull my day at work might have been, it is always immediately made better by coming home to a welcome like that.

I ask Leah how her day in school was and she mentions that she'd complained to her teacher about her back being a little sore. I ask her if it is still sore now. She says it isn't. I give her a good old-fashioned 'Dad bear hug' and she laughs. She can be such a drama queen sometimes.

Friday 16th November 2018

I received a call at work today from one of the paediatric consultants. He is the clinical director for the women's and children's services at the Trust. I've worked with him and his management team in the past on one or two projects and they are a good bunch. Apparently, the business manager's job for the services is going to be advertised soon and he recalled me saying that I could be interested in giving it a go a while back. I went over to see him and to discuss the potential opportunity over a coffee. It sounds like a really interesting role and I leave the conversation quite excited about possibly giving something brand new a try.

When I get home from work later in the evening, I speak to Claire about the meeting I'd had and the possible new job opportunity. Claire knows me well enough to know that I need a new challenge every now and then to keep me busy. I know how much I drive her insane because I can never sit still, but she's learned to put up with me over the years. She says she will be supportive if I decide it's what I want to do. This is a big relief, if I'm honest, because I've already pretty much decided that I should give this a go.

Later on, I go into Leah's room to tuck her into bed and say goodnight. We start chatting, as is the usual ritual when she is desperately trying to get another ten or fifteen minutes before lights out. During the conversation, she mentions that her back had been sore again in school today. Specifically, when she was sat on the floor in class with her classmates while the teacher read to them. She says her teacher had allowed her to sit on a chair as a one-off and that had seemed to make it better for her.

'That's good,' I say to her. 'It sounds like you've hurt your back playing and you maybe need to just rest it a little until it gets better?'

'Yes, I think so, Daddy' she says.

'Goodnight, darling. I love you. Sweet dreams,' I say as I turn her light off.

'Goodnight, Daddy, I love you plus one,' she replies, the same as she does every night.

'Plus one' is something that comes from Claire's family, but the girls have really latched onto it, especially Leah. Whenever someone says, 'I love you', the reply was always 'I love you plus one'. This means that even if I was to say 'I love you millions', the reply of 'plus one' would always represent one more. One more than any number I could say. It's really cute and it has become a bit of a catchphrase for our whole family.

Me being super-competitive, I respond to Leah with: 'I love you plus two'. This is instantly shot down, though, as it is apparently 'against the rules'.

'Against the rules plus one!' I say and strut out of her room with a smug grin on my face.

'Dad, you're such a loser,' is the faint response I hear as I close the bedroom door.

Saturday 24th November 2018

Saturday is now firmly 'football day' for Leah. We have a well-rehearsed routine for getting her kit on, packing her football bag and driving to football practice before 11am. The journey to football is only ten minutes in the car, but during the journey I notice that Leah isn't sitting straight in her car seat. When I ask her why, she says her back is sore again. This 'on and off' sore back has been going on for a couple of weeks now. It doesn't seem to be showing any signs of going away on its own so I'm starting to get a little concerned.

When we get home from football, I mention it to Claire. She says that she has also heard Leah complaining of a sore back on a couple of occasions over recent weeks. We agree to keep an eye on things and stop her from doing anything too strenuous for a week to see whether that sorts the problem out.

Saturday 1st December 2018

No football today for Leah as kicking a ball around a football pitch with a group of girls definitely counts as strenuous exercise. However, despite her more relaxed regime, the on/off issues with her back seem to have persisted. Claire and I have agree we need to get her examined at some point soon to see if she's damaged her back in some way. Claire decides to take her to the local walk-in centre later that day.

At the walk-in centre, Leah is seen by a nurse practitioner who feels her back and asks her a few questions. The result is a clinical opinion that she's probably just strained a muscle in school and we should give her Calpol and refrain from any exercise for a few days.

It is a relief to hear that she hasn't done anything serious, although that is what we expected to hear them say. She is constantly up and about and playing out with her friends, and I'm certain she wouldn't be so active if she'd done any serious damage to her back. Always helpful to get that reassurance, though.

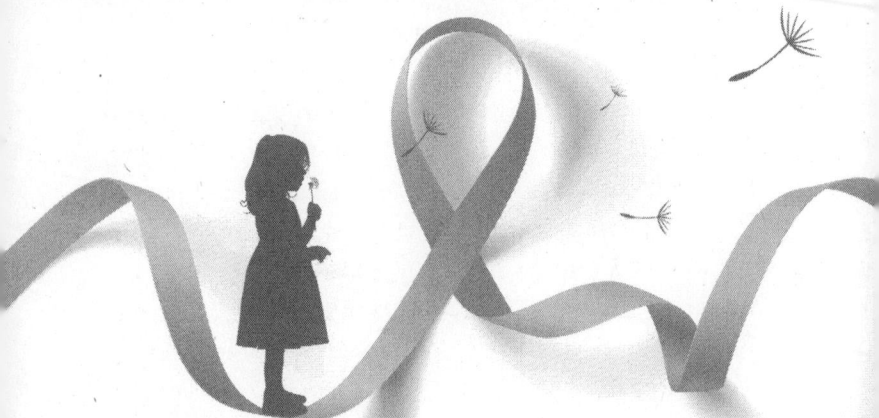

Leah Lemon

The time is just before 1:30pm on Wednesday 22nd August 2012. I'm stood in delivery room seven on the birth suite at Whiston Hospital in Prescot. My knuckles are white as my hand is being squeezed in boa constrictor-like fashion by Claire. In contrast, her face is bright pink. Her hair is stuck to her forehead with sweat. She looks totally exhausted. I've been told many times in the last twenty minutes that this situation is all my fault. I'm not in a position to argue right now.

Claire looks at me with a slight look of resignation on her face.

'One more, baby. You can do this. One more big push and you're there,' I say to her like I do this every day.

The midwife stood at the business end has adopted the 'catch it' pose as if she's a fielder playing cricket. We're all set.

Claire visibly feels the next contraction and, with one more huge effort and a guttural screech (from Claire, not me), out pops the star prize – 7 lb 13 oz of perfection. Weird, freakishly bluey-purple perfection. Time stands still while the whole room waits for the noise. Within a couple of seconds, the baby lets out a cry, which is the unofficial signal to say, 'Don't worry, I'm okay.' The relief is immense and the emotion and adrenaline of the last few hours now turns to tears that roll down my cheeks.

The midwife smiles and proudly lifts the baby up, unglamorously displaying the nether regions to me. I stare between the baby's legs for a few seconds. My head is hazy and I can't quite compute what is happening.

'It's a girl, Mr Bennett,' she says with a smile and a slight eye roll. 'Congratulations.'

'Oh yes. Thank you,' I respond. 'It's a girl, Claire! We've got another girl!'

Claire is just staring at me; her expression says it all: 'No shit, Sherlock.' Leah Grace Bennett has just become the fourth (and final) member of our perfect little family.

As time passes, it becomes more and more clear that Leah is very different to her older sister, Phoebe. Phoebe is often quite shy, quite timid, a little nervous and anxious about new situations. Leah, on the other hand, has a confidence beyond her years. Determined and fierce, but with a good sense of humour and a level of natural empathy rarely seen in a child of her age. The character differences between our two girls becomes increasingly visible as they grew up together.

We take them to a Little Mix concert in Manchester

in 2018 and the group ask the crowd if anyone would like to come up on stage and sing with them. I look at Phoebe. She is hiding under her seat, completely mortified about the thought of being picked. I glance across at Leah. She is stood on top of her chair, frantically waving her arms and shouting to be picked. We are in the cheap seats up in the gods, so she has no chance, but it doesn't stop her trying.

Leah had a pale-yellow T-shirt that she used to wear when she was younger. A few of my family started to call her 'Leah Lemon' whenever she wore it. She liked the nickname. It made her smile and it kind of stuck with her for a couple of years.

Leah is a really unique little lady. She is always very comfortable in her own skin and doesn't really pay too much attention to what others say or think about her. The second she comes home from school, she strips out her hair bobbles and clips, kicks off her shoes and does her own thing. I love that about her.

She loves to sing and dance, but she never knows the song lyrics and she's far from the world's best dancer. Does she care, though? Not one bit! Little did we know as she was growing up that her tenacity, determination, spirit and downright sass would play a key role in her future.

Throughout her life, Leah has had many different responses to the classic question: 'What would you like to be when you grow up?' From a vet to a nurse and a hairdresser to a footballer. However, the one response that often recurs is: 'I want to be Hermione Granger'. I, for one, certainly wouldn't bet against her achieving it. I'm just waiting for an owl to drop off a letter.

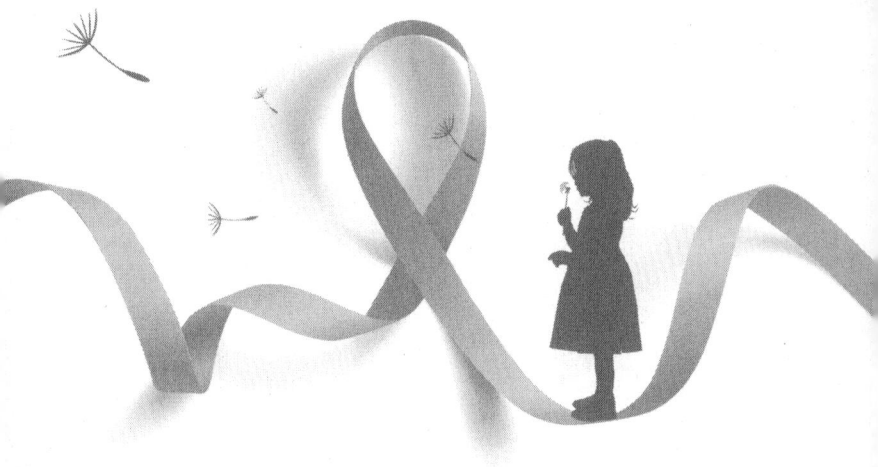

Hogmanay

Christmas 2018 has been and gone in a flash. The girls got completely spoiled, as always, by both mine and Claire's families. This year, there seems to have been a definite shift away from the pink plastic rubbish they seem to get every year towards electronic gadget-type toys. A welcome move in my eyes. Especially because no one seems to have noticed that Leah's brand-new tablet computer has miraculously come preloaded with the latest edition of *Grand Theft Auto* (more #DadSkills).

We usually alternate spending Christmas Day between my family and Claire's. However, since Marie's diagnosis, spending Christmas anywhere other than with Claire's family is not really an option. We spent Boxing Day with my immediate family at my mum and dad's house, and the day after, packed up the car and headed up to Scotland. Claire's family own a holiday home on the beautiful Isle of Bute and we try to get there a few times a year. This time, Claire's mum and dad, and her sister, Amy, and her family are coming up with us. We're planning to stay until the New Year (or Hogmanay, as it immediately becomes known the moment you reach Gretna).

We are about twenty minutes into the journey up the M6 when I notice Leah is sat slumped over in her car seat. When I ask her why, she says her back is sore again and she can't sit up straight. I glance at Claire and Claire glances back at me. We are both thinking the same thing… why is she still saying her back is sore? We are just going to have to keep an eye on her again during the week. It is already looking like a trip back to the walk-in centre when we get home.

The ferry crossing over to the island is a little rough due to the weather and the forecast for most of the week didn't look great. The house is a sanctuary, though. A warm and cosy place not only away from the Scottish island weather, but also from the pressures and challenges of normal life.

We arrive at the house in the late afternoon and it is already dark outside. Claire's mum and dad arrived a few hours earlier. Stepping through the front door, the feeling of warmth hits me immediately. The smell of dinner cooking in the kitchen wafts down to the front door. When I walk into the front room, I see they have put the Christmas tree up in the bay window and it looks amazing illuminated against the darkness outside. Phoebe and Leah run straight to Claire's mum and give her the biggest hugs. Everyone is smiling and feels safe. I can tell from Marie's face that, for a moment, her personal struggles are a million miles from her thoughts.

The house on Bute is a really special place for the whole family. It is a place where we can always escape when life gets tough. It connects Claire's family to previous generations, who travelled 'doon the watter' from Glasgow and the surrounding areas for holidays many years ago. Marie, herself, holidayed on the island as a child.

We stay at the house for just under a week, during which we get out onto the beach with the dog and play games round the kitchen table, and the girls go out trekking on horses. There is always a warm mug of hot chocolate on offer and an opportunity to bake cakes or shortbread. It is a place – *our* place – to spend good old-fashioned, wholesome family time. It is always hard to jump back on the ferry and leave it behind.

Across the week, Leah seems okay. She enjoys the pony trek and is happy running round on the beach despite the cold weather and drizzle. The same can't be said about Marie though, unfortunately. As the week goes on, she really struggles to get out of bed in the mornings. There are a number of occasions when I hear her vomiting in the bathroom in the early hours with Peter comforting her. It is really tough to see her struggling so much, but she is a determined lady and she gets up every morning and joins in with the day's activities.

We set off for home on Wednesday 2nd January. The day is another bank holiday in Scotland as they have two.

Based on the noise from the local pubs at Hogmanay, I suspect the extra bank holiday is being used to sleep off the hangovers. Leah again travels home lying across the back seat as her back is uncomfortable.

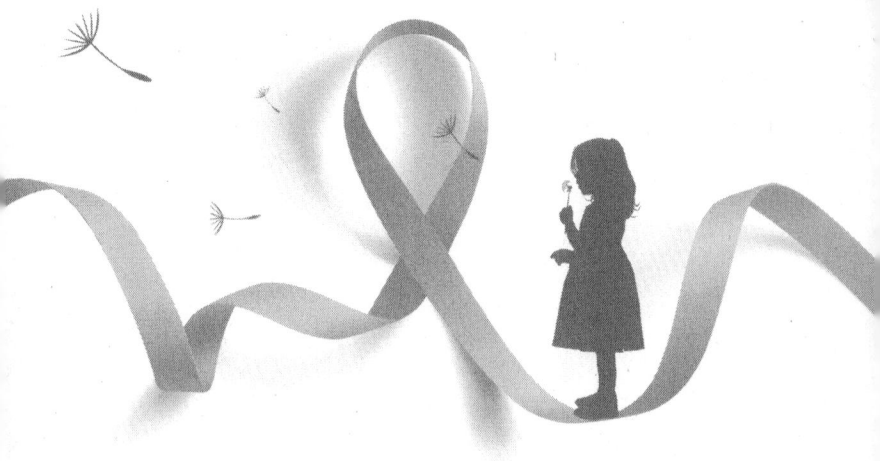

The Calm Before the Storm

Friday 4th January 2019

It is my first day back in work after Christmas and I have been given some good news... I've been offered a six-month secondment in the business manager job that I enquired about back in November! I'm thrilled to get the chance to do something new. It's a brand-new challenge for me and I can't wait to get started working with the women's and children's teams in the hospital. I'll be starting on the February 1st, so less than a month away.

Sunday 6th January 2019

One of the girls' Christmas presents from my mum and dad was a voucher for a skiing lesson at the Chill Factore in Manchester. Neither of them has ever tried skiing, so it's a new experience for them and they are both looking forward to it (Leah slightly more than Phoebe, if truth be told).

Leah doesn't quite hit the age range for the older children's group, so she is put in a group with the younger ones, while Phoebe goes with the older group. I watch them both closely from across the other side of the training slope. Within an hour, Leah is flying down the little slope, bending her knees with her arms stretched up over her head and a huge smile across her face. I take a photo of her and send it to my mum to say thank you for the vouchers.

Phoebe is far less 'gung-ho' about the experience and takes a little longer to relax and get the hang of it. By the end of the session, though, she is snow-ploughing slowly down the slope and I even see her smile at one point. Perhaps we'll get away for our first ever family skiing holiday next winter? Now, that would be exciting.

Thursday 17th January 2019

It is my birthday. The ripe old age of thirty-eight. We always do something small to celebrate every birthday we have in the family, so we decide to go out for dinner after work/school as a treat. I ask the girls where they want to go. Immediately, in unison, they both say their favourite Chinese restaurant local to where we live. They both love Chinese food. I should clarify at this point that both of them agreeing to the same thing without first having a huge argument/fight/period of intense negotiation is a rare occurrence.

We sit down and order a banquet meal for the four of us. Leah seems tired and I notice that she's a little pale in colour, too. She can often be like this towards the end of the week after a few days in school, so it doesn't concern me hugely. However, she also doesn't seem to have much of an appetite this evening and she doesn't eat much of the banquet. The fact that the basket of prawn crackers survived says everything because that is almost unheard of.

Claire feels her forehead, but she doesn't feel particularly hot to the touch.

'I think you might be coming down with a little bug, Leah. Do you not feel very well?' Claire asks her.

'No, Mummy, I feel okay. I'm just a bit tired,' Leah replies. As soon as the meal is finished, a cake is brought out and the girls blow the candles out[1] on my behalf. After that, we pay the bill and head home to get Leah to bed.

Just before midnight, there is a shout from Leah's bedroom on the top floor of the house.

'Mummy. Daddy. I need you!' I quickly jump out of bed and run upstairs to see what the matter is. Leah is sat upright in her bed with her bedside lamp on and a pile of vomited rice and noodles all over the bed and the carpet. 'I've been sick. Sorry, Daddy,' she says timidly.

'Oh, don't worry, baby. You clearly have got a bit of a tummy bug, haven't you?' I reply. 'I can clean it up. You strip those dirty pyjamas off and go down and get in bed with Mummy.' She does just that as I start stripping the

---

1 'Blow the candles out' – aka deposit half a pint of aerosolised saliva all over Colin the Caterpillar's back legs.

bed sheets and trying my best not to vomit myself in the process. Happy birthday to me!

Friday 18th January 2019

Claire and I have agreed to keep Leah off school today as she clearly wasn't well last night. She slept in our bed no problem after she'd recreated the scene from *The Exorcist* last night, and she was as bright as a button when she woke up. We kept her off school regardless and she was absolutely fine all day. It must have just been one of those twenty-four-hour things, I guess?

Saturday 26th January 2019

We sent Leah back into school last Monday and she has been great all week. So much so that she has asked whether she could go back to football today. I agree to take her as she does seem to have shaken off whatever illnesses and ailments she's had over recent weeks.

The girls do their usual training session and towards the end of the session, they all split into two teams and play a small match. It makes me smile so much watching them playing, having fun and enjoying themselves. Leah plays really well and makes some great passes to her teammates, even setting up one of her team's goals. She plays so well, in fact, that her coach awards her the trophy for 'Player of the Day' and the smile on her face stretches from ear to ear.

However, the smile on Claire's face is less enthusiastic when Leah gets home and shows her the ridiculously oversized trophy she's won, which is now going to take pride of place on the mantelpiece for the rest of the week.

Sunday 27th January 2019

Leah woke up feeling great again this morning, so to give Claire a bit of peace for a couple of hours, I take the girls swimming. Leah swims a full length of the pool without any help, which is the furthest I've ever seen her swim on her own, and she manages it really well.

In the evening, I make chicken and rice for dinner – two of Leah's favourite foods. I put the girls' plates out first and shout them down to come and eat. They both start tucking in, but very quickly Leah puts her knife and fork down and says she doesn't want any more. She has barely touched the plate. There are some foods that we constantly try and encourage Leah to eat. She can be a bit fussy on occasion and she refuses to even try many of them. Chicken and rice, however, is never a challenge and she will usually happily scoff the lot (and more).

When I asked her why she doesn't want it, she puts her head on the table as if completely exhausted and tells me she isn't hungry and has a sore tummy. Immediately, Claire and I are both concerned about her again. Something just isn't right and it's been going on for a while now.

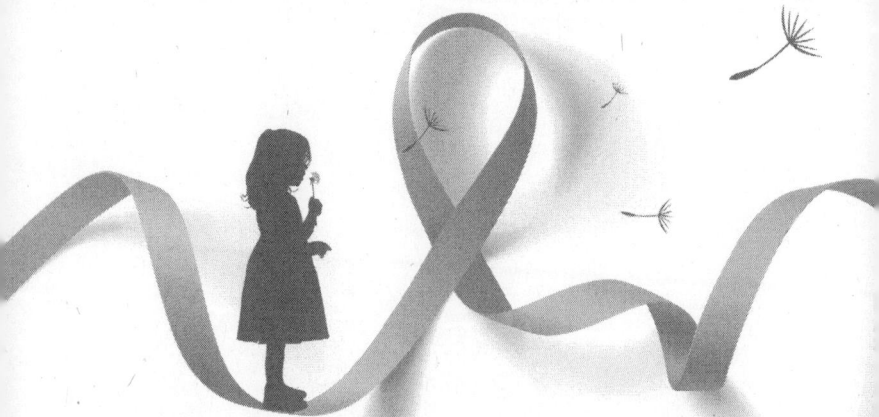

Lovely Dianne off the Telly

Claire and I are sat in the living room in the evening of Wednesday 30th January 2019, watching TV. *The One Show* is on. They have just finished an article about pineapples and they are about to launch into a feature about dog grooming. Save me now!

My total lack of interest in dog grooming (or pineapples, for that matter) makes my mind wander. I start browsing through the BBC News website on my phone and I come across an article about the BBC North West tonight weather presenter Dianne Oxberry. Dianne tragically lost her life to ovarian cancer a few weeks earlier after being formally diagnosed just a matter of days before.

Claire asks me what I was doing.

'Nothing, I'm just reading the news on the BBC website,' I reply.

'Anything interesting?' she enquires.

'Just an article about that lovely Dianne Oxberry off the telly.'

'Ahh, it's so sad, isn't it?'

The article includes a small footnote listing the symptoms of ovarian cancer. I start to read from the list:

- Feeling full quickly and/or loss of appetite
- Extreme fatigue
- Pelvic or abdominal pain

As I'm reading the words, my heart feels like it stops for a moment. I read them again. And then again.

These are things that we've noticed in Leah over recent weeks. She's been off her food, even her favourite foods. She's been really tired – at times that have been unusual. She's complained about pain in her back. I know that's not really her pelvis or abdomen, but it still makes me worried. There is clearly a connection between some of the specific symptoms and some of the things we've observed in Leah.

Oh God…

What if?

Surely not!

No, of course not. Don't be so stupid.

I calm myself down and convince myself I'm just overreacting. There are, after all, a number of other symptoms also listed that I definitely couldn't relate to Leah. *Stop this, Stephen.*

I'm clearly overreacting. In fact, I'm being ridiculous. Even so, I can't get the thought out of my head. It's planted itself in there now. I suspect no amount of trying to convince myself I'm being stupid is really going to override it.

Later that evening, I share some of my concerns with Claire.

'I'm worried about Leah; she just doesn't seem right. She's been tired and off her food for a few weeks now. Do you think you could call and get her an appointment with your GP in the morning? We should probably get her checked out... just to play it safe.'

I don't tell her about the article. I don't dare. She'd be absolutely out of her mind with worry. Besides, it's just me overreacting, isn't it?

Claire agrees that it is probably the right thing to do. 'Okay, I'll call them tomorrow and see whether I can get her an appointment and see what the GP says.'

I decide it is best to keep my worries to myself with this one and we go to bed for the night.

I barely sleep a wink.

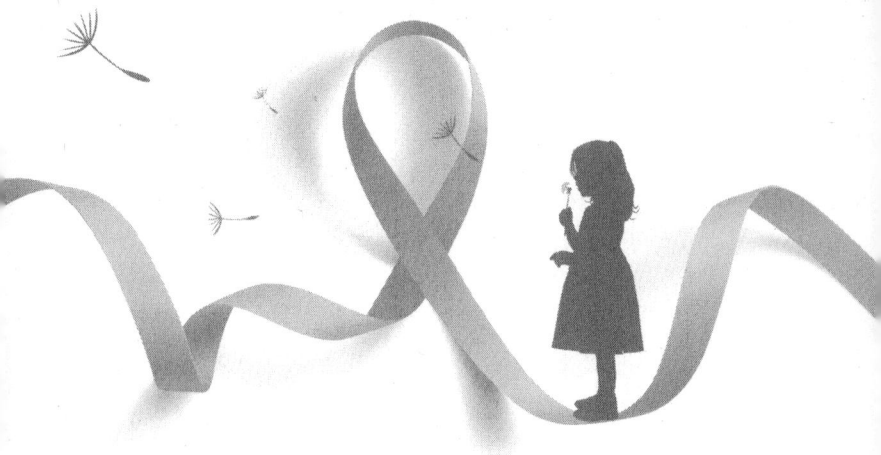

Jelly Pots and Piss

Thursday 31st January 2019

My drive into work this morning is dominated by anxiety. I can't stop thinking about the article I'd read the night before. I'm certain I'm worrying over nothing, but every time I push it to the back of my mind, it fights its way back to the front quite quickly. Claire is calling to get a GP appointment later this morning. If there are any genuine concerns, we'll soon have her checked out again.

She calls me at 9:30am to tell me the earliest she is able to get Leah in to see the GP is Tuesday next week (5th February). This isn't the response I was expecting. The article I had read last night has sent my head into a spin and it's made even more difficult because I can't really tell anyone about it. The thought of having this all racing through my head for another five or six days is simply unbearable. I really need someone to tell me she is okay and that I'm being silly to think otherwise.

I tell Claire that I don't really want to wait until next Tuesday, so I will speak to someone in the paediatric service at the hospital and ask if they can get someone to check Leah over if I bring her into work. I contact the team as soon as I put the phone down on Claire.

'Just bring her into PAU (Paediatric Assessment Unit) after lunch and we'll get one of the consultants to review her' is the answer I get. Phew! At least I can stop panicking.

I call Leah's school and inform them that I am coming to collect her to take her for a hospital appointment. I leave work straight after lunch, drive to Leah's school to pick her up and then drive back to work with Leah and take her straight to PAU.

When we get there, it is quite quiet and we are shown straight to one of the six bed spaces on the ward, only one other of which was occupied. They are clearly expecting us because they seem to be familiar with mine/Leah's name when we give it.

Leah is asked to give a urine sample while we are waiting for the doctor on duty to come and review her. She is clearly a little unsure about whether to get the sample alone or take me into the bathroom with her[2], but eventually she sheepishly asks for my help and we find the nearest facilities.

I have been given what can only be described as a relatively shallow empty jelly pot and I'm wearing a fairly

---

2   Even at six and a half years old, it is clearly not cool to have to pee in front of your dad.

smart two-piece suit. I'm already trying to work out the logistics of how this is going to work without me getting covered in it. After five minutes of pretty embarrassing and slightly undignified manoeuvring, we have a small amount of urine collected in the pot... and a lot more soaked into the sleeves of my suit.

After the ordeal with the sample, we return to the bed space. Leah jumps on the bed and lies down. She is really chatty and bubbly. I'm already starting to regret bringing her in and wasting the time of the staff. Not really the greatest first impression of the new manager, is it? However, I was... *I am* genuinely worried about her, so I know I've done the right thing bringing her in. Even if they tell me there is nothing wrong with her, at least we can all stop worrying, right?

About half an hour later, the doctor comes onto the ward area and smiles at us.

'Leah Bennett?' she enquires as she pulls the curtain around the bed space. 'Hello, Leah, I'm the doctor on duty today. Is it okay if I examine you and ask you a few questions?' Leah nods her approval coyly and relaxes back on the bed. The doctor asks Leah lots of questions as she feels her abdomen.

'Is there any pain when I press here?'

'How have you felt at school today?'

'When was the last time you went to the toilet?'

'Have you been eating and drinking okay?'

I explain to the doctor that she generally seems fine most of the time, but for the last month or so, she just hasn't quite been herself. She has complained of discomfort in her back and more recently in her tummy and she's been a little lethargic and off her food, but nothing has really been consistent. I'm almost apologising already for wasting her time.

'I can feel something in her abdomen,' the doctor says. 'But I suspect she just really needs the toilet, especially if she hasn't been for a few days. I don't think it is anything to be concerned about.' She prescribes Leah a gentle laxative. She is to take three sachets of the stuff with water every day for the next few days and see whether things improve. She also advises us to keep Tuesday's appointment with the GP in the diary in case we have any further concerns or we don't see any improvement before then.

The sense of relief is just immense. However, it is coupled with a sense of embarassment as I feel that I've wasted their time bringing Leah in and also allowed myself to get so distracted by something that turned out to be, literally, a load of shit!

We collect the laxative from the hospital pharmacy on the way out and then pop by my new office to say hello to a few of my new team. Leah takes great pleasure in spinning round on the swivel chair in front of my new desk[3]. I feel the knot untie in my stomach and breathe a huge sigh of relief. I also realise that my sleeve still stinks of piss.

---

3   By 'new desk', I do – of course – mean new for me. Not new as in brand-spanking new. I have mentioned that I work in the NHS and therefore the desk looks like it has been used by the KGB, a number of tax officers, Henry VIII and Noah on his ark at some point during its extended life.

Friday 1st February 2019

Today, I officially started my job as business manager for women's and children's services. I'm excited about the new challenge and raring to get going. My day was mostly spent handing over the duties of my old role and speaking to the senior members of my new team. I feel fresh and energised and super-keen to do my best and try to make a positive impact on the services.

Saturday 2nd February 2019

Leah has been so much better today. The laxative seems to be doing the trick, although I have been watching her trips to the bathroom like a hawk since Thursday. I have to say that I haven't noticed anything out of the ordinary. She seems to have been going quite regularly and she's told me that she's emptied her bowels, so hopefully we'll see her starting to pick up properly now. She went to football today, as the usual Saturday routine dictates, and she seemed okay running around with her teammates. All the signs are good again.

Sunday 3rd February 2019

I wake up in the morning and Leah is bright and chatty. Claire gives her another sachet of the laxative just after breakfast and she drinks it down as normal.

We go out for Sunday lunch with Claire's family to our favourite restaurant in the town centre. Leah has a beautiful white frilly lace dress on. She looks super cute. We all sit down and Leah starts to colour in a picture that one of the waiting staff have given her with a small pack of crayons. She still looks a little pale to me, but she orders chicken nuggets from the children's menu and a glass of apple juice, and sits there colouring away. Leah loves chicken nuggets and I mean *loves* them, so this will be another interesting test of how she is feeling. If she doesn't eat these, then we can safely say something still isn't quite right.

Everyone's starters arrive and are eaten. Leah looks really tired and I notice she has stopped colouring in and is laying her head on the table, looking really lethargic.

'Are you okay, sweetheart?' I ask her.

'Yes, Daddy, I'm just really tired,' she replies.

A few minutes later, the main meals arrive at the table and the young waiter places a tasty-looking plate of chicken nuggets with chips and peas down in front of Leah. I watch her covertly from across the table as she picks up her fork and stabs a nugget. She takes a really small bite, then puts the fork down and puts her head back on the table. I try to encourage her to eat and ask whether she wants me to cut her food up for her. 'I'm not hungry' is her response and she is genuinely disinterested in her meal. My heart sinks. This is just not like her.

When we get home from the restaurant, Claire and I agree that we need to keep the GP appointment booked for Tuesday and take her along as planned.

Monday 4th February 2019

Today is the start of my first full week in my new job. I spend the whole day meeting other members of the team, attending meetings and setting up all my personal belongings in my new office. Ballpoint pens, highlighters, a decent stack of Post-it notes and a couple of boxes of Cup a soups (for the inevitable 'lunches on the go' that seem to have become the required cuisine of choice for the NHS manager over recent years).

Pride of place on the desk next to my PC monitor is a framed photo of my two girls. A picture taken by Claire of them stood hugging each other in the bandstand at a local park a year before. They both look happy, but freezing cold. The picture makes me smile. Like many people, I like to have a photo of my kids on my desk for a few reasons. Firstly, it's always a good talking point when meeting new people. Secondly, it reminds me exactly why I'm sat doing the job during those moments when you start to question yourself. Speaking of which, I found out that I'm down on the rota to do my first shift as site manager on Wednesday (shadowing one of the other managers). Talk about being thrown in at the deep end! I'm a little nervous about this, but excited in equal measure.

I don't get a minute all day to worry about Leah, but Claire is taking her to see the GP tomorrow anyway so nothing will change until then. Fingers crossed they can finally prescribe something that might help her bounce back to her usual self.

Tuesday 5th February 2019

Another busy day in work today filled with lots of meetings of questionable importance and far too many emails! Claire doesn't work on a Tuesday so she is taking Leah to see the GP straight after picking her up from school. I have a meeting in my office to discuss the staffing levels on the paediatric ward at 4pm. There are four of us (including myself) huddled round a small corner table, poring over numerous printed spreadsheets and staff lists. Fifteen minutes into the meeting, my mobile goes off in my pocket. I pull it out and glance down at the screen. It's Claire.

I excuse myself from the meeting temporarily and go outside to take the call. Claire sounds quite agitated.

'Hi, honey, it's only me. Listen, we're on our way to A&E at Whiston. The GP has sent us.'

'A&E?' I say, slightly alarmed. 'Why A&E? What's the matter with her?'

'He doesn't know, but he examined her tummy and he doesn't like it, so he's sent us to A&E for further examination.'

'Okay,' I say, trying not to seem too flustered, 'I'll leave work now and meet you there.'

'Great. My mum and dad have got Phoebe, so don't worry about her. Just call me when you get here and I'll tell you where we are'. I take a second outside the office before walking back in.

'Really sorry, folks, but I'm going to have to go. My daughter has been sent to hospital and I need to go and join my wife.' Immediately, everyone agrees to call a halt to the meeting (sensing I am a little worried) and swiftly leaves the room. I shut down my computer and leave work to meet Claire and Leah at Whiston Hospital.

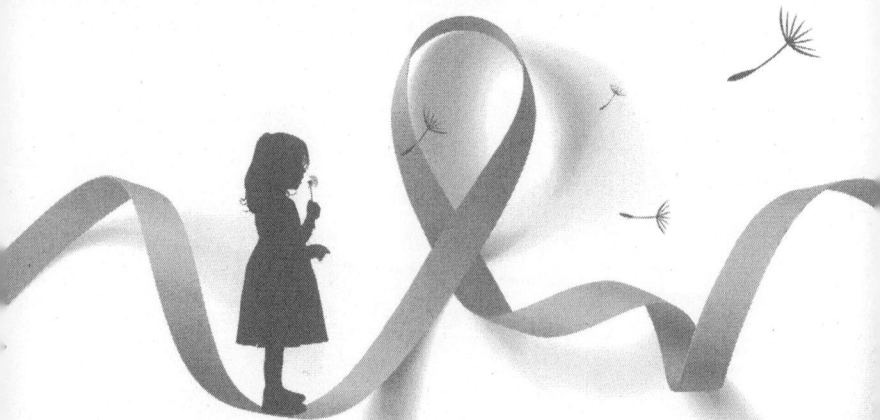

The Beginning of the Rest of Your Life

I call Claire when I arrive in the hospital car park and she tells me that they have already been transferred up to the children's ward. Leah has just had a blood sample taken by a relatively junior doctor and, by all accounts, it didn't go well. Apparently, the doctor was quite nervous and struggled to find a suitable vein in the back of Leah's hand. Eventually, after a few clumsy attempts, he succeeded, but just as he inserted the needle, Leah looked down at her hand and pulled it away, spraying blood all over the bed she was sat on (and presumably all over the doctor, too). It sounds like it was a fairly distressing experience for all involved, so I park up my car and hurriedly make my way to meet them on the ward.

When I arrive at the ward, one of the nurses asks who I am here to see.

'Leah Bennett – I'm her dad,' I say. She looks at me with a kind of knowing look as if she had anticipated my words, then she shows me round to the room at the end of the main corridor in the corner of the ward. Inside, Claire is stood up at the foot of the bed that Leah is lying on. She is still in her green school uniform, but with a small bandage over her left hand following 'bloodgate'. She greets me with a big smile and a 'Hi, Daddy!'. She looks really bright, alert and perfectly well. I immediately feel less anxious.

I kiss Claire on the head and give her an attempt at a smile. I can see she is worried. Her eyes say everything about how she feels.

'Have you seen her tummy?' Claire says to me. I shoot her a puzzled look and she stands over Leah on the bed and lifts up her polo shirt. The reason for the GP's concern is immediately apparent. I freeze on the spot. On the right-hand side of her abdomen is a large and very visible lump. It's about the size of a small orange. I am absolutely stunned. What the hell is this and how has this just seemingly appeared overnight? She was checked over at another hospital last week while I was stood there and this... this... *thing* was definitely not there! My initial shock quickly subsides into terror and my heart is racing. I am so scared. I know that I have to force myself to remain calm so as not to worry Leah. I can tell Claire is thinking and feeling the exact same things as I am. We don't even need to talk about it; we both just know that this is way more serious than we imagined even this morning. I don't think either of us truly believes this is constipation anymore, but I also don't think anyone has wished for something to be true so much in their life.

Over the course of the next few hours, one by one, progressively more senior medical personnel come into the room to speak to Leah, to us, and to check and feel her abdomen. A nurse, then a more senior nurse, then a junior doctor, then a specialist nurse, then a middle-grade doctor and eventually a consultant. Leah is chatting away to one of the healthcare assistants, who is helping her to draw round her hand and colour it in. I am beside myself with worry, constantly telling myself not to overthink things and remain calm. Eventually, the specialist nurse, a lovely lady called Jackie, comes back in to break the news that they plan to keep Leah in hospital overnight to run more tests on her. I agree to stay in with her, so Claire goes off to fetch me some fresh clothes and toiletries from home, before picking Phoebe up from her parent's house and returning home.

Leah and I start to settle down for the night and I send my work colleagues a text message. I'm fairly certain I won't be doing that on-call shift tomorrow now.

Wednesday 6th February 2019

It took me a while to get to sleep last night. So many questions and worries flying through my head. Eventually, and probably through nervous exhaustion if nothing else, I dozed off. At around 1am, I get tentatively awoken by another of the healthcare assistants, who has come on duty for the night shift. He politely asks whether I could rouse Leah to take her down to radiology for an X-ray.

'What? Now? At this time?' I ask.

'Yes, if you can,' he replies.

Leah is fast asleep, so she takes a while to come round, but (reluctantly) agrees to come down for the X-ray with me. Walking through the hospital in the early hours is quite a spooky experience. The usual spaces that are bustling with staff, patients and visitors during the day are now deserted, dark and eerily quiet. The X-ray is done in a matter of minutes, and Leah and I return to the room and go straight back to bed. It takes me a lot longer than Leah to fall asleep again.

When we wake again later that morning, Leah gets a bowl of Rice Krispies from the housekeeper who is doing the rounds with the breakfast trolley. She sits up in bed and has a few spoonfuls, but quickly decides she's had enough and pushes the bowl to the side. I'm watching what she eats so closely now, desperate for any sign that her appetite might be returning and that she is picking up.

Claire phones to check how she was overnight and tells me she is going to drop Phoebe off at school and then make her way back to the hospital later in the morning. She has already phoned Leah's school to tell them she won't be coming in today.

At around 11am, the consultant on duty that day, Dr Udasi, comes into the room with her team to review Leah. There are at least four people with her. Leah is lively and chatty and doesn't look as if there is any reason for anyone to be concerned. I am sat at the end of the bed. Leah lies down and pulls up her pyjama top so that Dr Udasi can feel her abdomen. There it is, staring back at me, this big lump that has seemingly just appeared out of nowhere.

Dr Udasi produces a measuring tape from her pocket and starts to measure the dimensions of this lump with the help of one of her colleagues. I hear her state that it is around 12cm wide. She turns to look at me and says, 'I'm pretty certain this is not a faecal mass.' I didn't really need her to say this – in my heart, I already knew – but at that point the realisation of how serious this is hits me like a train and I become overwhelmed by the situation. I start to become distressed. I just can't hold back the tidal wave of emotion and tension I feel. I break down in tears. Jackie, who is in the room with us, spots me and escorts me out, so as not to upset or alarm Leah. She takes me to an empty room down the corridor, gives me some tissues and tells me to use the phone in the corner of the room if I need to call anyone. I know Claire is already on her way back into the hospital and there is nobody else I needed to call, so I just sit and sob for five minutes. Soon after, Claire arrives and is shown into the room with me.

She immediately runs to me and throws her arms around me.

'What is it, Ste? Where is Leah? What's up with her?'

'She's in the room and she's okay,' I reply through the tears.

'What's up then? What's happened?'

'Nothing,' I say, 'but they don't think it is simply constipation anymore.'

'What the hell is it then? Oh God!' Claire says, now just as distressed as I am.

I just shrug. I don't know the answer and I'm not

sure that I want to know it either. The body language of everyone around us suggests this is serious, but we haven't had any answers yet. My brain is jumping all over the place and my heart is racing. Based on Claire's reaction, I think she also knows this is something serious, but has been trying not to let those thoughts in.

After a couple of minutes, we both compose ourselves enough to go back into Leah's room. The medical team have now left and she is sat up playing with one of the hospital play specialists. She has a small figurine of Elsa from *Frozen* in her hand and she is chatting to the play specialist about trainers. By coincidence, they happen to have the exact same pair of trainers (albeit different sizes, I must add!) and Leah thinks this is cool. The play specialist has completely distracted Leah from the situation and she is blissfully unaware of the terror that is unfolding around her. It is a beautiful snapshot in what now feels like a war zone.

Around an hour later, we are asked to escort Leah back down to radiology again, this time for an ultrasound examination. Leah is in a chair pushed by a porter and we are accompanied by one of the nurses from the ward. We are stood in the corridor outside the ultrasound room, waiting. Leah is chatting to the nurse, and Claire and I are just stood hand in hand watching them. Every so often, one of us will just squeeze the other's hand a little tighter as if to say, 'I'm right here and we've got this'. I feel a little sorry for the nurse stood with us, firstly because Leah is talking non-stop to her about some random TV programme she'd seen recently and she can hardly get a word in edgeways.

But secondly, because she has no idea what to say to Claire and I. How could she? Surely they don't encounter these situations every day. Surely they don't train hospital staff how to converse with parents who are worried sick about what is happening to their child. Do they? If they don't, maybe they should. In fairness, I'm absolutely not in the mental space for a good conversation, and I don't think I would absorb anything she said at that point anyway. She tries her best to give us reassuring smiles every so often and it is appreciated nonetheless.

We eventually go inside the room and the ultrasonographer greets us and tells us his name. He could have told me his name was Queen Elizabeth and I wouldn't have remembered it. The nurse is also in the room with us.

Queen Elizabeth picks up the scanner handpiece and covers it with a blue gel. Leah takes off her pyjama top and he places the handpiece onto her abdomen. She recoils slightly because the gel is cold on her skin. The room is dimly lit with the main light coming from the screen of the scanner. It is really hard to decipher what it is I am looking at on the screen and, in the end, I stop trying. Instead, I turn my attention to the ultrasonographer and I watch his facial expressions as he scans Leah's tummy, taking little screenshots of what he can see at regular intervals. There is a real sense of tension in the room and the body language of everyone inside suggests that there is a lot of concern all round. I am desperately trying to pick up some positive signs from anywhere, but there aren't really any to be found.

After the ultrasound, we go back up to the children's

ward and take Leah into the playroom. She wants to do some colouring, so she sits down at a small plastic table with a pot of colouring pencils in the middle. In typical NHS fashion, most of the pencils are snapped and/or blunt, but between the three of us we manage to scrape a basic selection of colours together. She picks up a pile of prints and rifles through them to find a picture to colour in. She chooses a Christmas elf.

'Christmas was ages ago, sweetheart. Why have you picked an elf?' I ask her. I look through the rest of the pile of prints; a Christmas tree, Rudolph the red-nosed reindeer or a Christmas pudding are the alternatives she could have chosen – bearing in mind it is early February. Never change, NHS, never change.

Leah sits and colours in the elf picture for twenty minutes or so with a little help from Mum and Dad[4]. We are about to turn our attention to a small plastic guitar on the opposite side of the room, when the play specialist comes in and offers to play with Leah for a while. Behind her is Jackie, who beckons Claire and I over and then asks us to come with her. We follow her down the corridor and she stops at the ward manager's office, opens the door and then ushers us inside, closing the door behind us.

The office is narrow and has a long worktop down one side with a couple of PCs on it. Around the walls are lots

---

4   Leah must have coloured in 200+ pictures while at nursery/ school and our fridge door is usually covered in some of them before they mysteriously disappear after Claire or I have a good kitchen clean session. I've kept that Elf picture and I still have it to this day. It's crazy what becomes precious to you all of a sudden following difficult experiences.

of laminated posters and box files on shelves, and a very faint smell of coffee wafts through the air. Sat at one end of the room is Dr Udasi and she has one of the paediatric specialist nurses stood behind her. Jackie is stood behind us in front of the door. Directly in front of us are two empty chairs. Dr Udasi invites Claire and I to sit in them. My heart is thumping out of my chest. I am absolutely terrified. I imagine it is like kneeling in a guillotine waiting for the blade to drop.

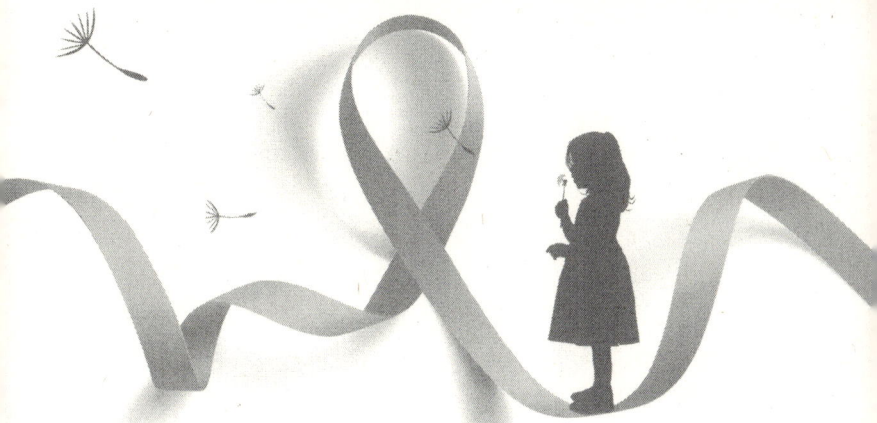

Breaking News

Wednesday 6th February 2019 (cont'd)

Nobody speaks for what feels like an eternity. My eyes are darting between everyone in the room, hoping to pick up some sense of what is about to happen. Nobody meets my gaze. They are all looking at the floor, ashen-faced.

Dr Udasi then breaks the silence. She says *those four words*.

'We think your daughter may have a tumour, perhaps a carcinoma or a sarcoma. I'm so, so sorry.' She looks emotional as she says the words to us. Her words seem to hang in the air and then echo off the walls around us. I'm staring at the faces around the room again. They are all now wide-eyed, close to tears and stood like cricket fielders, poised and ready to catch us or scoop us up from the floor.

There is a harrowing silence for a few seconds in the suddenly claustrophobic room. The silence is then broken.

'No!' shouts Claire. 'That can't be right! Not my daughter as well as my mum!'

I feel empty. I feel helpless. I feel like I want to shout out with every joule of energy my body can muster, but I can't. I'm paralysed. It all feels hazy and blurry – like an out-of-body experience. I feel the tears building up in my eyes and then I feel a comforting hand on my shoulder from one of the nurses stood behind me. This is real. This is not fake. I can't hold the tears back anymore. Claire and I both break down and just sit there, holding each other in sheer disbelief.

Between them, the team try to explain that they are speaking to Alder Hey Children's Hospital in Liverpool to arrange an onward referral and they ask whether we need anything. They agree to leave us for a few minutes to gather our thoughts and try and scrape ourselves up from the floor.

We sit there in the empty room for ten minutes or so. We just hold each other. Clinging on. Shaking our heads in denial. How can this be true? The room feels like it is closing in around me. I need to get out. I desperately don't want to leave Claire and I don't want anyone outside this room to see me, but I cannot stay in here. I tell Claire that I need to go and speak to my mum.

'Don't leave me. Please don't leave me,' she says.

'I have to get out of this room, Claire,' I beg.

She looks me in the eye and solemnly nods her

approval. I feel terrible leaving her here, but I cannot stay in the room for another second.

'Please can you call my mum?' she asks. 'I can't speak to her right now, but please ask her to come in.'

I leave the room with my mobile phone in my quivering hand and walk into the nearest side room, closing the door behind me.

Inside the other room, I sit by the window and stare out for a minute or so. How the hell do you ever prepare yourself to make a phone call like this? What on earth do you say? I decide to call my mum first. I think that might be the easier call. I ring her mobile. She is out at the shops, but she answers immediately. She knew Leah was in hospital and she will have been desperately waiting on my call.

'Mum,' I say, my voice already quivering. 'They think Leah has cancer, Mum.' She pauses. I can hear the shakiness in her voice.

'Oh God. I'm coming in now. Where are you?'

Immediately after I end the call to my mum, I know I have to make the call to Claire's parents. This is the one I am dreading the most.

I call Marie's mobile and she, too, answers immediately. She will sense my voice is cracking straight away, so I just spit out the words.

'Marie, they think Leah has cancer.'

It's the most difficult thing I've ever had to say in my life.

'No!' she says. 'God, no! This cannot be! I'm so sorry, Ste. I'm so sorry!' The raw emotion in her voice is audible.

I hear Marie turn to Peter and tell him the news and then the anguish in Peter's voice in the background. Marie agrees to come into the hospital with Peter and we end the call. The tears stream down my face once more.

After a few minutes, I compose myself slightly and go back into the ward manager's office. Claire is sat in the exact same position that she was when I left the room. Jackie is now sat next to her, holding her hand, and she is cradling a small plastic cup of water that I assume Jackie has brought her. As I walk in, Jackie greets me with a compassionate smile. Claire and I sit for a few more minutes, just throwing questions into the air... How? Why? When? No answers come back.

Twenty minutes later, we make our way back into the room at the end of the corridor and sit down on some plastic chairs in the corner, holding one another. Soon after, there is a knock on the door and my mum tentatively walks in. She walks straight up to me and throws her arms around me, with tears running down her face.

'I'm so sorry, Ste.' She then hugs Claire so tightly I think she's going to fracture her ribcage.

I need some water so I leave the room to get some. As I walk out, I bump into Marie and Peter, who have just walked onto the ward. As soon as they see me, they both break down.

'I'm sorry, Ste, so sorry. This shouldn't be happening.' They hug me tightly. I show them into the room where Claire and my mum are talking, and both run up to Claire and hold her so tightly. The five of us are now together in the room, every one of us broken into a million pieces.

Everyone is desperate to go and see Leah, so again we compose ourselves and go back to her room around the corner. She is sat on the bed playing with the *Frozen* dolls with the play specialist, without a care in the world. With a painted smile and a broken heart, we each kiss her on the cheek and join in with her game.

An hour or so later, the ward manager comes to see us with some information that he thought might be useful. He hands me a paper booklet he has printed off the internet. It is entitled: 'My Child Has a Kidney Tumour' – or something along those lines. At that moment, I can't imagine I will ever have the strength or focus to read it, but I thank him anyway. He clearly just wants to try and help in some small way. He brings us back into the end room along with Dr Udasi and they tell us they have referred Leah onto Alder Hey. We are told to report to Ward 3B first thing on Friday morning, where they will pick up Leah's care. In a daze, we gather together Leah's belongings and head home.

On the way home, I message work: 'I won't be doing the on-call tomorrow. In fact, I don't think I'll be back for some time.'

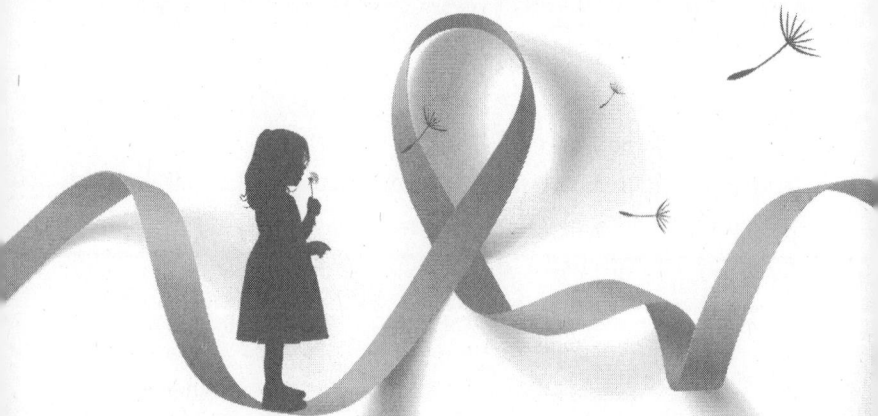

What? How? Why?

Thursday 7th February 2019

I hardly slept a wink last night. Neither did Claire. A constant cycle of fear, hope and confusion ran through my head on a seemingly endless loop.

Why her?

Why us?

Why not me instead of her?

We are having to deal with this with Claire's mum; it's just not fair that we now have to deal with it with Leah, too! Surely that's not fair.

How did we not spot this earlier?

How did others not spot this earlier?

When will her treatment start?

What will that mean?

How do we tell Phoebe?

What about school?

What about the holiday we've just booked?

What about work?

Does she have a chance of surviving this?

If not, how long has she got?

What the actual fuck is a carcinoma?

Plus another million questions... going round and round and round as I lay there in the dark, without knowing any of the answers. It was absolute torture. Our near-perfect world has been shattered and, all of a sudden, we are lost. Surrounded by darkness. So scared.

Friday 8th February 2019

Friday morning comes round and we take Leah to Alder Hey as instructed. Inside, I'm still clinging to a faint hope that we will find out that the team from Whiston have, in fact, made a mistake and this is not what we fear it is. Leah is allocated one of the beds on the oncology and haematology day care ward (Ward 3B). Claire and I pull up chairs and sit down beside her bed, still feeling dazed and completely lost. Leah is clearly apprehensive about what is happening. I have no doubt she can also sense the fear oozing out of Claire and I, despite our best efforts to keep it hidden.

Over the course of the morning, Leah is examined by a number of the medical team and we are asked many questions. In particular, lots of questions about our family history and whether cancer is prevalent in either of our families. Claire describes to the team that her mum has been diagnosed with renal cancer and is currently receiving treatment. I can see it is painful for Claire to even talk about.

Early that afternoon, we are asked by the nursing team to take Leah down to the radiology department for an MRI scan. The purpose of the MRI scan is to obtain a more detailed picture of whatever is inside Leah's abdomen in terms of both the size and the position. Everything about the scan is new to Leah, as well as Claire and I. She is nervous, but she comes downstairs to the radiology department with us.

The MRI scanner is a large and fairly daunting piece of equipment. Leah is greeted by a lady called Debbie, who is running the scanner that day. Debbie invites her to lie down on the table at the mouth of the machine. She is really friendly and chats to Leah, as well as to us, and she works some magic by putting Leah at ease. However, Leah is still quiet, and clearly nervous and unsure about what is about to happen. Once Leah lies back on the table, Debbie packs a number of foam wedges around her to restrict her movement while she is inside the scanner and places a large panel over her chest, which plugs into the machine. Finally, a mirror is mounted over Leah's head and a large pair of headphones placed over her ears. She looks like some kind of trainee astronaut as she slowly disappears inside the machine.

Claire and I sit at the foot of the scanner, staring into the tunnel so Leah can see us throughout the scan. We are given headphones, too, as the noise from the scanner is loud. Leah has chosen a film to watch on the TV during the scan and we can just see her eyes reflecting in the mirror above her head, through which she is watching the film. She looks tiny and vulnerable inside this huge machine and the fear in her eyes is hard to ignore.

The machine kicks into life and the noise is loud. It sounds like an eighties' prog-rock synthesiser turned up to full volume. As soon as the scan starts, I glance over at Claire. She is praying. I have never really felt any benefit from prayer personally, but it feels like we need all the help we can get right now, so who am I to question it?

After about twenty-five minutes, I notice Leah's eyes starting to well up with tears and I can see that she is trying to tell us something. The noise of the machine and the headphones mean that I can't hear what she is saying. She also can't really move, so she seems unable to point out what is wrong either. A couple of minutes later, Debbie notices Claire waving and pauses the scan. She comes back into the room and withdraws Leah from the tunnel. She is crying at this point and Claire and I rush to her to find out what is wrong. The earphones she is wearing have folded one of her ears over and it is causing her pain. She didn't want to move to fix it as she had been told to remain as still as she could for the scan. We fix the headphones properly back over her ears and she calms down quite quickly, before being returned to the machine to complete the scan.

The scan lasts around forty minutes in total. When it is finished, Debbie returns to the room and withdraws Leah from the tunnel once more. Debbie's body language seems different now; she has a slight look of melancholy and she is certainly less chatty with us than she was before the scan. I try not to read too much into it. Debbie informs Leah that she needs to inject some dye into her arm in order to take the final few scan pictures. Leah gets distressed at this suggestion. When she realises this will require a needle into the back of her hand, she refuses point blank. I'm guessing that her extreme reaction is partly linked to the blood sample debacle at the previous hospital.

After a few minutes of us all trying to persuade Leah to agree to do it, Debbie decides not to distress her anymore and agrees not to continue with any further scan pictures. Leah gets off the scanner in double-quick time before she changes her mind and we take her home. She doesn't talk to Claire or I for the whole journey home.

Saturday 9th February 2019

I set up a new WhatsApp group today called #TeamLeah and added all of mine and Claire's immediate family into it, so that we can share news with them all simultaneously. I'm really conscious that I have a ton of unread and unanswered texts and WhatsApp messages on my phone from people who have heard the news about Leah. People must be being kept informed via our families because I don't feel like I've spoken to anyone else other than Claire and the Alder Hey staff for a lifetime. I know that people want to know what is going on and want to help us, but I just haven't had the strength to go through the messages and I've got even less strength to respond to them. I pluck up the courage to post something on social media to avoid having to reply to all the messages individually. Within a couple of hours, the responses to the post has topped the one hundred mark. Every single one so supportive and heartfelt. They bring me to tears.

On a less positive note, Leah's physical condition seems to be starting to deteriorate. She seems to be in a lot more pain and discomfort with her back than ever before. She is now routinely struggling to sit upright in a chair for more than ten or fifteen minutes.

This nightmare is getting more and more real, and more and more difficult. I have no idea if, when or how this is going to end, but I do know for certain we have an army of support behind us already.

Sunday 10th February 2019

We've been invited round to my mum and dad's house for dinner with my sisters and their families. Mum loves having the whole gang around and today it feels extra special given the events of the last week. I'm not sure whether I am mentally ready to see everyone together with Leah in the same room, but the feeling of warmth and love engulfs us all as soon as we walk in and I immediately feel more comfortable.

The conversations stay clear of getting into too much detail and negativity, especially when Leah is around. Instead, everyone is treading a narrow path between wanting to provide a helpful distraction and a dose of normality, while also acknowledging that they are concerned and really wanting to help us. It is a strange and unfamiliar atmosphere that I've never experienced in my parents' house. I sense the underlying pain and emotion, and I sense even greater the desire to support and that alone is helpful in a tiny way.

We are all sat round the table and Mum and Dad start bringing out a number of steaming hot bowls from the oven, containing the component parts of a lamb Sunday roast. Leah is sat at the head of the extended table, but is not looking comfortable. After several attempts to adjust her sitting position with various cushions from the sofa, it is clear that we are not going to be able to find a suitable solution that will allow her to sit in these high-back, upright chairs and eat her dinner. Claire takes her over to the sofa in the adjoining living room and makes her comfortable in a position where she can lean back slightly and take some of the pressure away from her lower back. This seems to do the trick and she seems to settle down. She is then able to eat a small amount of food with Claire sat next to her for company.

As soon as others finish their dinner, they immediately move into the living room and join Claire and Leah. I look across at my dad. Tears are streaming down his face. He is trying not to make it obvious that he is upset. This is really hard to see and it dawns on me that this is perhaps the first physical sign of Leah's deteriorating physical state that those close to us have seen. My dad is so upset and can hardly speak – the reality of just how serious the situation is has started to hit home for everyone.

Monday 11th February 2019

We're heading back to Alder Hey for further tests, reviews and examinations. We will also get to meet the consultant who is taking over Leah's care today. His name is Professor Barry Pilling. I never met Barry during my time working at Alder Hey, although I heard his name in a number of forums. It is quite a surprise to meet him in the flesh and he looks totally different to what I expected. He is short with glasses that sit on the end of his nose and he approaches Leah's bedside on day care dressed in a poorly fitted black suit and a pair of black training shoes. He seems like an eccentric character and certainly not what you might expect a consultant paediatric oncologist to look like.

Barry introduces himself to Claire and I and spends a few minutes chatting to Leah and examining her abdomen. Around twenty minutes later, he returns and asks Claire and I to follow him into one of the consultation rooms next to the ward. Cautiously, we enter the room. Inside, there are two other men. One is introduced as one of the oncology registrars (senior doctors training to be consultants) and the other as Dr Hanley, a consultant interventional radiologist.

Barry starts off the conversation by cutting straight to the chase. He confirms our worst fears. Leah has a large malignant tumour – she does indeed have cancer. The tumour has seemingly grown from one of the bones towards the bottom of her back and grown forwards into her abdomen. I suppose it is what we were expecting to hear, but the words still hurt.

Barry then describes the immediate plan for Leah to us. We need to bring her back into the hospital on Wednesday to go to theatre where Dr Hanley will be available to take biopsies[5] of the tumour. The biopsies will be sent to the laboratory for analysis in order to help provide a formal diagnosis of Leah's condition and subsequently inform a treatment plan for her. It feels like a lot of information to take in and I still feel in a slight daze with the whole situation. It still doesn't really feel real.

Dr Hanley then describes how the procedure on Wednesday will work. Essentially, they will punch into the tumour from two points at the base of Leah's back and extract the biopsy samples using a needle. I have to ask for a glass of water at this point. I feel very close to passing out. This is just a complete nightmare. All the time I am thinking about the horrible situation that my little girl is going to have to go through and how frightened she will be. I feel sick.

I know the people in this room with us mean well and are offering to help us, but the whole conversation is very matter-of-fact. This type of conversation and the language used is clearly very 'normal' to these people, but I am completely lost, trapped in a terrifying world that I know nothing about and don't understand. Every word is like a hammer blow to my body or a dagger through my heart.

That night back at home, Claire and I decide not to tell Leah too much about her going to the theatre on

---

5   A biopsy is a medical procedure that involves taking a small sample of tissue from the affected area, which can then be analysed under a microscope.

Wednesday. We don't want her to panic and be frightened. She was extremely frightened about the prospect of getting a needle during the MRI scan the week before, so we agree it is probably best to give her the minimum information possible about what is to come. Time will tell whether that is the right thing to do or not.

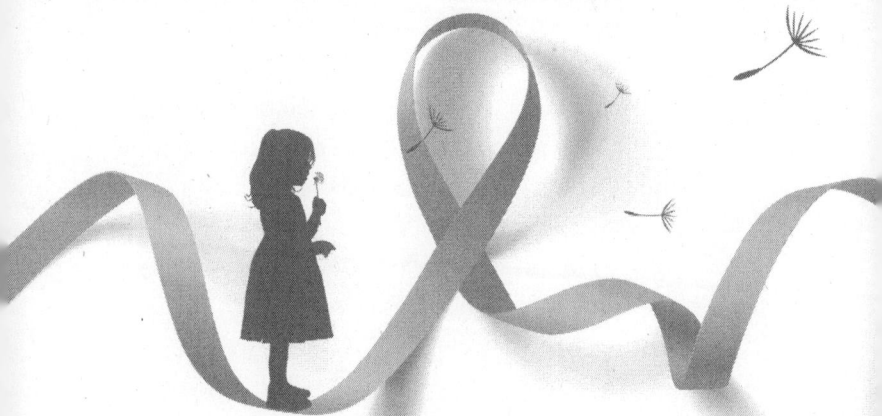

The Blob

Tuesday 12th February 2019

We are not required to go to the hospital today, so we have a chance to pause and reflect on the whirlwind events of the last week. Neither Claire or I have slept or eaten properly in that time. The strength of anxiety within us both has completely taken away our appetites and ability to switch off our brains and rest. We are both physically and mentally exhausted, and still haven't fully processed what is happening to us all. It is also the first time we have really had a chance to speak to each other about the situation.

Perhaps unsurprisingly, it turns out that Claire is in the same headspace as I am. She is struggling to process the amount of information we have received over recent days, and is continually asking herself how this has happened and why it might have happened to us. I don't know if we'll ever get the answers to those questions and I don't think it would change anything if we did. I constantly ask myself the same ones, though.

That night, we put Phoebe to bed in her usual room in the attic space of our house. Leah's room is opposite Phoebe's room on that top floor, but tonight we have agreed that Leah will sleep in our bed with Claire and I. She is struggling more and more with her back now and we feel that we need to be with her all the time. Phoebe is really unhappy at sleeping on the top floor alone. She says she is scared. I suspect this is less about being on the top floor of the house alone and more to do with the fact that she clearly knows Leah is not well and something is going on. We haven't told her any more details at this point. We don't really know that much more ourselves, to be honest. It's fairly clear that we're going to have to have that conversation with Phoebe sooner rather than later. The thought makes me sick to my stomach. We'll deal with that when the time is right. For now, she'll keep going to school and just know that Leah is a little poorly.

Soon after Phoebe has gone to bed, Claire and I go, too. Leah has already made herself comfortable in the middle of our bed surrounded by a mountain of pillows. After the usual hour or two of worrying, overthinking and questioning the world, exhaustion takes hold and I start to fall asleep. Leah is underneath my left arm in bed and is extremely fidgety. She is uncomfortable and she mentions that her back is sore when she lies flat on the bed. I move my arm position so I can prop her up slightly and take some of the pressure away from her lower back. This seems to do the trick and eventually she drifts off to sleep. The position I'm now lying in is really uncomfortable for me, but I don't dare move a muscle even though I can barely feel my arm. It must be around 3am before my brain finally overrides everything else and shuts down.

I wake up twenty minutes later with pins and needles in my left hand. I desperately don't want to move my arm. Leah is lying on it and she's asleep, pain-free and peaceful. Right now, I would cut it off myself if it meant she could lie there, dreaming.

Wednesday 13th February 2019

We're back at Alder Hey for the biopsy procedure. Before that, we are sent back to the radiology department for Leah to have a CT scan. Aside from the now usual battle to get her to agree to have a needle as part of the scan procedure, everything else goes smoothly. Getting Leah to agree to a needle has become a huge challenge for us already, but it is clear that this is something we are all going to have to get used to.

The afternoon soon comes round and it is time for the biopsy. It is going to be Leah's first ever trip to theatre and we have no idea how this will go. We are all apprehensive. We have told Leah that she has to go to theatre 'for tests', but she is unaware of exactly what that means at this stage (as are Claire and I, to a degree).

At around 1pm, the call comes from the theatre team for Leah to make her way over. We gather our belongings, help her off the bed and make our way out of the ward and down to the theatres. We reach the anaesthetic room and Claire and I are talking to Leah and trying to keep her spirits up. She is visibly nervous about what is to come. She has already told us that she does not want to have a needle, and we have calmed her fears by telling her that she doesn't have to have one and that she can choose to have some 'sleepy gas' instead. She is still unsure about it all, but the thought of perhaps having a less traumatic option seems to calm her immediate fears.

The anaesthetic room is small and there are a lot of people inside. Leah is clearly agitated and very frightened. The environment is daunting for her. The anaesthetist introduces himself as Dr Johnstone. He has a neatly trimmed beard, glasses and is wearing a bandana on his head instead of a theatre cap like everyone else in the room. He looks like a drummer from a nineties' rock band (except he is wearing theatre scrubs). Dr Rock God tries his best to calm Leah down and asks her whether she would like him to use the gas or a needle. Without a moment's hesitation, she opts for the gas and he passes her a small face mask connected to the anaesthetic machine. She holds the mask over her nose and mouth and takes a few breaths. I can tell she is unsure, but she seems relatively okay with it all. So far, so good, I think. Then Dr Rock God turns on the anaesthetic gas. Leah can smell or perhaps taste it immediately and straight away she starts to panic and pull the face mask away from her face.

'My head feels funny, Daddy!' she shouts, staring at

me, terrified. 'Mummy, help me! I don't like it!' I look at Dr Rock God and our eyes meet. He doesn't actually say anything, but the look in his eyes says, 'I'm really sorry about this, Dad, but you know we need to do it.' He then clamps the mask to Leah's face and holds the back of her head. She struggles a little, but then I watch as her eyes roll back and she falls asleep. Dr Rock God lies her back onto the trolley and it is done.

The whole ordeal probably only lasts around five minutes, but – my word – it is extremely distressing. Both Claire and I leave the room in tears. Outside, we are comforted by a member of the theatre team and told to go and get a drink. We'll receive a call when she is out of theatre and we can come back and see her.

An hour or so later, we get that call. Claire and I rush back to the theatre suite and we are escorted through to her in recovery. It is such a relief to see her. She is curled up in the foetal position on the trolley in the recovery area. I can see she has two large dressings at the bottom of her back on either side of her spine, on top of the orange stain of iodine.

She is still a little groggy from the anaesthetic, but she glances over her shoulder as we approach her. The first thing she says is, 'I hate you, Daddy.' It absolutely breaks my heart. She is obviously blaming Claire and I for putting her through this, but what choice do we have?

A couple of hours later, when Leah is fully recovered from the anaesthetic, we are told we can go home. We are asked to come back to Ward 3B in the morning for a few more small tests. We collect Phoebe from Marie and

Peter's house on the way home and we go to bed early, completely exhausted but totally unable to sleep. Again.

Thursday 14th February 2019

We are only required to take Leah to the hospital briefly today for a short ultrasound examination. We arrive home at around 2pm. Leah is really struggling to sit comfortably in any chairs in the house now and she is struggling more and more with pain in her lower back. The whole shit-show that seems to have become our lives for the past week or so has been beyond tough, but seeing my little girl in pain and suffering is just unbearable. Add to that the fact that I cannot really do anything to help her and it becomes absolute torture.

At around 7pm, the telephone rings and I answer it.

'Hello,' I say.

'Oh, hello, is that Leah Bennett's parent?' responds the voice on the other end of the line.

'It is – speaking,' I reply.

'Oh, hi, I'm really sorry to bother you and I'm not actually sure whether I should be making this call or not, but it's Jackie from the children's ward at Whiston. I just can't stop thinking about your daughter and your family, and I just wanted to check how you are all doing.'

I nearly drop the phone.

I give Jackie a brief update on what's happened over the last week or so. I also inform her that Leah is struggling a little and we're waiting desperately for her treatment to start. Jackie thanks me for the update, wishes Leah and our family well, and then ends the conversation by offering her help and support with anything that we might need. I thank her sincerely for reaching out to us and I tell her how much it means to us that people are thinking of Leah and sending their support. We then end the call. I put the phone down and break into tears, completely blown away by the sheer level of compassion and humanity that can be encapsulated by a simple two-minute phone call.

Later on, I am lying in bed in the darkness, staring at the clock on the wall. I realise today is Valentine's Day. It is the first time in nearly twenty years that Claire and I haven't given each other a card.

Friday 15th February 2019

We're back at Alder Hey for Leah to have yet more blood tests and ultrasound scans and to have yet more discussions with yet more clinical boffins. I'm losing track of who everyone is now and what purpose they serve. I haven't slept properly since last Monday. I'm still completely terrified – terrified that despite being told my child has cancer and despite her having been poked, prodded and scanned more than a discounted loaf of bread in Tesco, she still hasn't received any actual treatment that might help her.

All she has been prescribed so far is oral morphine (aka Oramorph) to help manage her pain, some anti-sickness medication (in case the Oramorph makes her vomit) and a medicine to help with constipation (a common side effect of Oramorph). None of that is actually doing anything to stop this bloody lump growing and taking over her body.

We are desperate for the Alder Hey team to finish all these tests and start her on some treatment as quickly as possible. Based upon how quickly she seems to be deteriorating now, it genuinely feels like she might not survive long enough to even have a chance of fighting back against this disease. Leah was skiing, swimming and playing football three weeks ago, and now she cannot sit in a chair or sleep without a dose of morphine. I'm struggling hard to stay focused and even harder to stay positive.

While on the ward, I grab the opportunity to put my fears across to Cat, one of the senior oncology registrars. I asked her for two minutes out of Leah's earshot and she agrees. We step away from Leah's bed and I essentially beg her to start some form of treatment.

'She is going to lose this fight without even throwing a punch,' I say to her. Cat explains to me that things are not that simple. They need to do everything they can to determine what type of cancer Leah has, as this will determine the most effective treatment protocol. I do understand this, but it is excruciating. My heart is breaking at the thought of losing my daughter without her even being given a chance.

After speaking to Cat, I walk back round to Leah's bed. As I get close, I can hear Claire on the other side of the curtain, singing 'You Are My Sunshine, My Only Sunshine' to Leah.

There are two nurses stood behind the desk opposite. They are both crying.

Monday 18th February 2019

The weekend passes without any major incidents. We are now managing the pain in Leah's back with regular morphine doses. Both Claire and I have spoken to our respective managers in work and brought them up to date with what is happening. It's safe to say that neither of our employers are expecting us back in work any time soon.

That afternoon, we are asked to go back to Alder Hey to see Prof. Pilling in clinic. He has received most of the results of the tests from the previous week and Leah's case has been discussed at the MDT[6] meeting earlier in the day. We are therefore hoping to find out exactly what we are dealing with, what the treatment plan will look like and, most importantly, when her treatment might commence.

We leave Leah on the ward with the nursing team and go across to the clinic room. Prof. Pilling wastes no time on pleasantries and jumps straight into the matter in hand. He proceeds to repeat the fact that Leah does have a large tumour emanating from one of the spinal bones in her lower back. He tells us that the MRI has shown that there is damage to the affected vertebral bone. He tells us that the tumour has started to envelope the organs and blood vessels in her abdomen. My mouth is dry at this point and my chest is aching. Every single sentence he says seems to take a bite out of my heart. He then turns around the

---

6   MDT stands for Multidisciplinary Team. An MDT meeting
     is where professionals with expertise in different aspects of a
     patient's care come together to discuss cases with the aim of
     reaching collective agreement on the best approach to treatment.

computer monitor on his desk to show us the MRI image.

Staring back at us from the large black screen is an image that will be imprinted on my brain for the rest of my life. It shows Leah's tiny body with an enormous white blob right in the middle of her abdomen. It takes a second for me to fully process the image in front of my eyes, but I quickly work out that I am staring at a picture of the tumour. The tumour that seems to be rapidly stealing my daughter's life from right under my nose. It is huge and ugly and evil. I close my eyes and try to catch my breath. The blob is still there. It is superimposed onto the back of my eyelids, akin to what happens when you stare at a bright spot for too long.

I open my eyes and lift up my head. Barry still hasn't turned the screen back and the blob remains there in front of me. I can see the extent to which her blood vessels are trapped inside it. I swallow hard, but my mouth is so dry. My heart is racing.

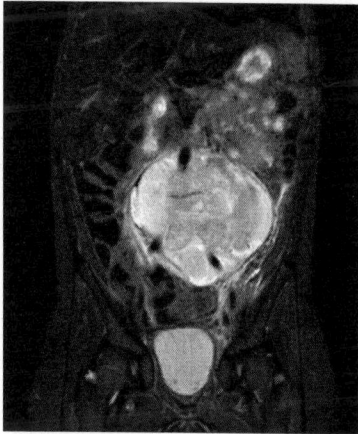

How the hell has she carried something that big around in her little body without us knowing? How long has this thing been growing inside her? How on earth is she going to survive this?

It is terrifying. My initial shock quickly subsides into a feeling of immense guilt and shame. I feel like I have let her down. Like I have failed her as a parent. I should have seen this sooner. I should have picked up on the signs earlier than I did. It all feels too late now.

I think back to Debbie in radiology and the look on her face when she completed the MRI scan. No wonder she seemed sombre when she came to get Leah out of the scanner. She had obviously seen this monstrosity appearing on the screen before her eyes and knew the scale of the challenge facing the little girl lying on the table on the other side of the glass.

The rest of the conversation with Prof. Pilling is a bit of a blur. He proceeds to tell us that they have not been able to profile the tumour against any recognised types of sarcoma, although tests are ongoing. Therefore, for the time being, it would have to be classified as an 'undifferentiated sarcoma' or an 'undifferentiated retro-peritoneal sarcoma' to be precise. This means that there is no obvious tried-and-tested treatment regime that is known to have any positive impact on the tumour. To make matters worse, the tumour has grown around Leah's aorta and iliac arteries, some of the body's major blood vessels. This means any surgical intervention to remove it will obviously be extremely risky.

Following wider discussion at the MDT meeting and

with paediatric oncology colleagues from other hospital trusts, Prof. Pilling has already taken the decision to commence treatment for Leah as soon as possible rather than delay any further. This was the only positive note from an extremely difficult and emotional fifteen-minute meeting. Positive in the sense that she might actually get the chance to fight back against this monster. Not positive in the sense that she is going to have to face gruelling cancer treatment. Christ only knows whether she has any chance of surviving this.

Given that the tumour type is still unknown at this stage, the treatment protocol Leah will follow will be based upon what the team feel *might* be most effective. We are told that the first round of chemotherapy treatment will begin on Thursday and we will need to bring her back in before then to prepare her for the treatment and to get more details about the treatment plan.

'Do you have any questions?' Prof Pilling asks.

I can hardly breathe or think straight, never mind ask any questions. I shake my bowed head. With that, Prof. Pilling leaves the room and Claire and I just sit there alongside one of the nursing team.

In total silence.

Shell-shocked.

Broken.

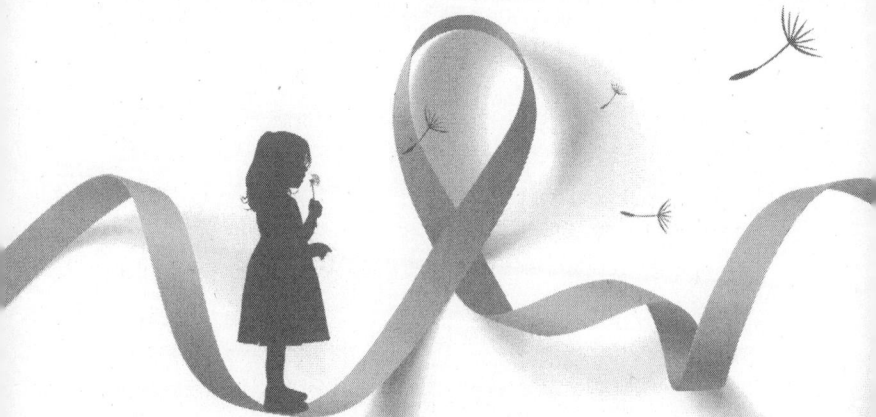

VDC-IE

Tuesday 19th February 2019

In order to have the chemotherapy treatment administered safely, and also to take regular blood samples without constantly having to jab her with needles, Leah needs to go back to theatre for the second time to have a central line[7] inserted. We have also been informed that she will get a PEG[8] feeding tube fitted during the same procedure. The PEG tube goes directly into her stomach and will allow us to ensure she receives essential fluids and nutrition in the event that the chemotherapy treatment makes her lose

---

7   A central line or central venous catheter (also known as a
    Broviac or Hickman Line) is a long, thin rubber tube inserted
    into a person's chest. It enters the major blood vessels near to
    or inside the heart and allows medicine to be easily delivered
    intravenously.
8   Percutaneous Endoscopic Gastrostomy.

her appetite or makes her mouth too sore to eat food – both of which are highly likely. We are starting to get some insight into how challenging the treatment might be for Leah, but we are still desperate for the chemo to start, just to give her that chance. We will all just need to deal with the implications after that.

Leah has been pencilled in for a slot on the emergency theatre list today to get the procedures undertaken. Being on the emergency list means that there is always a possibility of a higher priority patient taking precedence for the theatre time over Leah. This is out of our control, so we just hope she will be in and out as quickly as possible. Leah has not been allowed to eat from midnight last night and is also not allowed any fluids from 7am onwards.

We arrive back on Ward 3B day care at 8am and Leah is allocated a bed. We are told by the ward team that they are hopeful that she will go down to theatre around 11am, so she grabs her little tablet computer out of her bag, chooses a film to watch and then settles on the bed for a couple of hours. She is obviously nervous about going back to theatre, and Claire and I have discussed it with her to try and calm her nerves. She is refusing to have the 'sleepy gas' this time based upon the traumatic experience from the previous week. Instead, she reluctantly agrees to have a cannula inserted in the back of her right hand.

11am creeps up on us and we are told that another poor child has been taken into theatre unexpectedly as they have been deemed to be a higher priority than Leah. It is now looking like she will go to theatre in the early afternoon. She is allowed a small drink of water.

Just after lunchtime, Prof. Pilling comes to the ward to speak to Claire and I. We follow him down the corridor and into a small room on the main ward, where we are joined by one of the oncology outreach nursing team – a friendly, grey-haired lady called Michelle. For the next twenty minutes or so, Prof. Pilling explains the plan for Leah's treatment in more detail.

The plan is for her to receive regular rounds of chemotherapy treatment over an approximate nine-month period. At some point, the chemotherapy will pause and Leah will hopefully have surgery to remove the tumour. After that, she will undergo a course of radiotherapy at the Clatterbridge Cancer Centre over on the Wirral. Following successful completion of the radiotherapy, the chemotherapy will recommence. After a few 'stupid' questions and some points of clarity, I manage to ascertain that essentially the plan is to give her high-impact chemotherapy with the aim of shrinking the tumour significantly in size. This will hopefully move the tumour away from the major organs and blood vessels, which will make the surgery more straightforward. The surgery will then remove a significant proportion of the tumour and increase the chances of the subsequent radiotherapy treatment being effective. The radiotherapy will then aim to kill off any remaining cancer cells in Leah's body and the final doses of chemotherapy will help ensure that all cancer cells are killed off to reduce the possibility of the cancer returning.

The chemotherapy treatment protocol that Leah will receive is abbreviated to VDC-IE and will consist of five different drugs: Vincristine, Doxorubicin, Cyclophosphamide, Ifosfamide and Etoposide[9]. She will be given the VDC drugs across a three-day stay followed by a two-week gap. After which, she will be given the IE drugs across a six-day stay. There will then be another two-week gap before the cycle starts again.

The meeting with Prof. Pilling is tiring and we have to absorb an awful lot of information within a short space of time again. Her treatment is going to be lengthy and intense and that is difficult to comprehend, but at least we now have a plan. She's almost made it into the ring, ready for the fight of her short life.

In addition to explaining the details of Leah's treatment plan, Prof. Pilling also gives us the details of what to expect in terms of side effects. He starts to explain and I brace myself for impact. Claire is holding my hand and her knuckles are almost white from gripping so tightly.

'Okay, so she *will* lose her hair,' he says. Not 'she might lose her hair' or 'there is a chance she *could* lose her hair'. No. 'She *will* lose her hair… and that will start a couple of weeks after her first chemotherapy treatment.' His words again hit me like a punch in the face.

'It's very likely that she will get ulcers in her mouth and perhaps in her bottom.' Punch number two.

---

9   Cyclophosphamide is the oldest of these drugs and was developed in 1959. The youngest of these drugs, Ifosfamide, was developed in 1987. I find it gobsmacking that we are still treating some forms of childhood cancer with first-line treatments that are over thirty years old, when technology and medicine has progressed so far in that time.

'She will feel sick, probably very sick at times... but don't worry, we'll prescribe some anti-sickness medication for that.' Punch three.

'She probably won't want to eat much or perhaps won't be able to eat much after her treatment starts... but don't worry, that's why we're putting in the PEG tube.' Punch four. I'm on the ropes now.

'The thing I'm most worried about is her kidneys,' he continues. 'The chemo will damage them and it's highly likely that any radiotherapy she has will do further damage. It's also highly likely that she may need a kidney transplant at some point.' Punch number five and I'm down.

Sadly, these conversations must happen frequently in Prof. Pilling's world, and the way he states the facts as if reading from a textbook suggests this is not a new scenario for him. But for us, it is painful. Every word hurts. This is my daughter he is talking about. My little girl; my six-year-old little girl. And he's describing these utterly horrendous things that she's going to have to deal with as if they are football results or TV listings. We leave the meeting with the wind firmly knocked out of our sails. Left in no doubt whatsoever that the journey ahead of us all is going to be long and extremely painful.

We return to Leah's bedside, only to be told that it is now unlikely that she will go to theatre this afternoon as another child has taken priority. It is now almost 2:30pm and she has been frightened and nervous all day, and has not eaten a single bite of food. I am incredibly frustrated that she's had to go through this today – but, at the same time, I just want to take her home where she, and all of us, feel safe. None of us have the emotional energy to deal with a trip to theatre now. We pack up Leah's things in her bag and make our way home. Today has been tough.

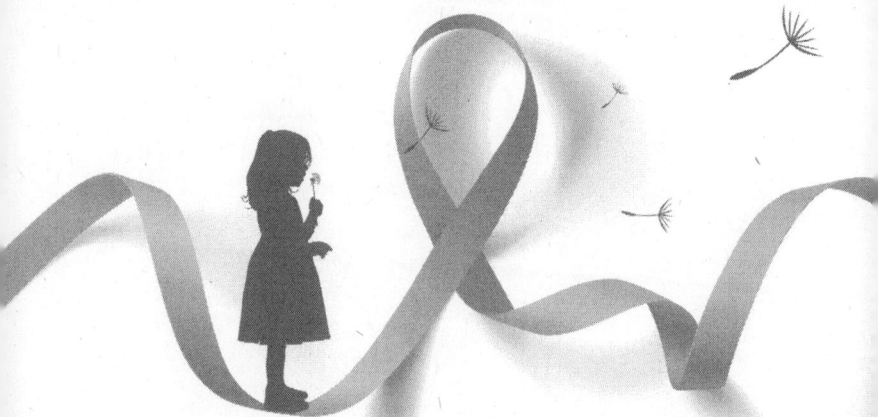

A Whole New World

Wednesday 20th February 2019

We're back at Alder Hey, hoping that we won't waste another day waiting for something to happen like yesterday. Thankfully, Leah gets her slot on the list mid-morning this time. She goes into theatre with relatively little distress (and without the sleepy gas) and we meet her in recovery an hour or so later, with the addition of a horrible white tube sticking out of her chest and another tube sticking out of her tummy. It is really hard to see her with these additions. I can't stop thinking about what her little body has already been through and will still need to go through over the coming weeks and months.

A couple of hours later, we leave the hospital. We collect Phoebe from my sister Debbie's house and return to the safety of our own home. Deb and her husband, Mike, kindly agreed to look after her for us today, which has been a big help. The girls go to bed early. Leah is particularly tired after another difficult day. Claire and I find ourselves sat in the living room together, alone for the first time in a while. We talk about today and we talk about our thoughts and feelings on yesterday's meeting with Prof. Pilling. It turns out Claire is really struggling with him. She finds his abruptness and bluntness really difficult to deal with. He is clearly a highly intelligent individual and undoubtedly a talented clinician in his field of expertise, but something is not quite working right now. We're going to need to find a way to manage his style of communication because it is creating a really negative emotional response, especially in Claire. We are both looking for positives and searching for glimmers of hope at the moment and we're not getting much from Prof. Pilling in that regard.

On the topic of communication, Claire and I discuss the fact that Leah isn't really talking to us very much right now. We suspect it might be because she is frightened and she probably senses that Claire and I are withholding information from her. We are beginning to think that keeping her in the dark about what she is going to have to go through is possibly not the right way to handle things with her. We agree that we have to involve her as much as possible in the conversations moving forwards, so she is more aware of what is going on.

Nobody tells you how to manage these situations. There is no guidebook. We're in a world that we know nothing about and we're having to learn from scratch. We're probably learning more at the moment through getting things wrong than getting things right. It is incredibly difficult. How do you even begin to explain to a six-year-old child that they are seriously ill and might not actually survive? How do you prepare them for the fact that the treatment they are about to face to give them a chance of survival will, itself, make them very sick and their hair fall out? How do we tell Phoebe that her sister, her best friend, has cancer? I honestly don't know where to start. I feel more and more lost every day.

Thursday 21st February 2019

Leah's first round of chemotherapy commences today, almost exactly two weeks after that fateful visit to the GP. The last two weeks of waiting have felt like an eternity, but I now have this strange mix of feelings to contend with. I'm immensely relieved that she is due to commence treatment, but, at the same time, I'm terrified about what lies in store for her and for the rest of us.

On reflection, it is quite astonishing that the NHS can test, diagnose and analyse for a condition like cancer, then formulate and prepare a treatment plan and insert the tools to administer that treatment all in less than two weeks. However, these have been the longest two weeks of my life. I just want it all to be over more quickly than it is taking.

We arrive on Ward 3B at 10am, carrying a carload of our belongings to help us get through the next few days. We've told Leah that she will be in hospital for three days while she gets the medicine she needs to shrink 'the lump' in her body. She seems okay with that as an explanation, so that's where we've decided to leave things for now.

We are on the inpatient side of the ward this time instead of the day case side, so it is all new to us. We are shown into a small bay of four beds and Leah has been allocated the bed in the far corner next to the outside windows. The bed opposite Leah's is empty. The two other beds are occupied. One has a curtain drawn all the way around. I can't see who is inside apart from through a small gap in the curtains, where I can see someone's knee in a pair of jeans. In the final bed, which is next to Leah's, there is a young boy, perhaps three years old, sat playing on a tablet computer. He is very pale in colour and has a tube running from behind his ear into his right nostril. The tube is taped to his right cheek. He has no hair. A dark-haired lady is sat on a chair next to his bed looking at her phone. She is mid-thirties in age. As we enter the bay, the lady glances up from her phone and gives me a sympathetic smile. She looks tired. I smile back.

One of the nurses on duty has been allocated the beds in the bay to look after today, so she comes and introduces herself to us all as Sam. She shows us where to put our belongings. There is a small chest of drawers, a narrow wardrobe, and a bedside unit for us to use to store our things. Sam then gives us a whistle-stop tour of the ward, pointing out the small parents' kitchen area, the small play area, the nurse's station, the side rooms, and the classroom. The classroom? It hits me for a second that Leah is going to miss an awful lot of school while she receives treatment, so of course there is a need for a classroom. Does this mean she will be far behind the other kids in her class when she finally gets through this and gets back to school? Brilliant. There is yet another daily worry that I'll no doubt have whizzing through my head at stupid o'clock each night. It's a fairly long list of worries now.

After the brief tour is complete, we return to the bay and Leah climbs onto her bed. One of the healthcare assistants on the ward called Neil approaches us and asks Claire what Leah's name and date of birth is. He confirms Claire's response against the info written on two coloured bands in his hand, then proceeds to place a band around Leah's right arm and another around her left leg. He shows Leah how to use the TV, which is fixed to a large metal arm on the wall above her bed. He then asks Claire and I whether we need anything. We say no and thank him.

At around 11am, Sam comes back to Leah's bed in the bay armed with a large tray of items including wipes, gloves and plastic packets with thin tubes inside. She is accompanied by another nurse called Jayne, who is carrying a small syringe containing a clear liquid, a large syringe containing a bright orange liquid, and what looks like a large bag of water. Sam tells us it is time to start the chemotherapy. The two nurses between them wheel a drip stand over to Leah's bed from the empty bed opposite. The drip stand has three small machines clamped to the central pole. Sam plugs the three machines into a bank of sockets located behind Leah's bed and they blink and beep into life.

Sam and Jayne check the names on the two syringes against Leah's wristband before hanging the bag of water on the drip stand and connecting it to one of the machines further down. The small syringe with the clear liquid is placed into a second machine and the large syringe containing the orange liquid is placed into the third machine. Sam types some numbers into the machines as Jayne shouts them out and the machines beep and flash in response. Jayne then connects the tubes from the machines to the central line tubes that are coming out of Leah's chest and releases the clamps on them. Sam presses one final button on each machine and that's that. The chemotherapy treatment has started. I feel relieved, but anxious in equal measure. For the next three days, Leah is going to be connected via a network of plastic tubes to the machines on the drip stand, which will slowly push the chemo drugs into her body.

Phoebe is on half term from school this week and has been taken off to Blackpool for the day with two of our close friends. I agree to stay in the hospital with Leah tonight and eventually Claire leaves the ward at around 7pm to collect Phoebe and go home.

Just before he finishes his shift, Neil pops in to see us and shows me how to set up my bed for the night next to Leah. The bed pulls down from the wardrobe unit in the wall. It is a single, wipe-clean mattress in a frame. Neil finds me a couple of thin pillows and shows me where to get bed sheets from a trolley on the main corridor. I walk over to one of the small bathrooms in the opposite side of the bay to brush my teeth before settling down early for the night. Leah is already asleep. I lie there on the mattress wrapped in a thin sheet. It is so cold next to the window. As I shiver, I also sob quietly to myself for at least an hour.

Friday 22nd February 2019

The overnight stay in hospital was tough work. The nurses were popping in to see Leah to check her temperature, blood pressure and oxygen levels every few hours. Also, Leah woke up and needed to use the toilet a couple of times in the night, so I had to help her out of bed, unplug the machines from the wall and then push the drip stand across the bay to the bathroom in the corner. Add to this the incessant beeping noise emitted by the machines every time Leah rolled over in her sleep and accidentally blocked one of the tubes, or when the syringe or saline was empty, and it meant there was little opportunity for sleep.

At 8am, Claire calls me to check how Leah is and how we'd got on overnight. I explain that neither of us slept very well and Claire immediately volunteers to cover the night duty tonight so that I can rest. I gratefully accept the offer. Claire tells me that she has already agreed to drop Phoebe off with her parents today and then she will make her way into the hospital.

She arrives on the ward at around 11am armed with an overnight bag for herself, some sweet treats for Leah and a large latte for me, which is also gratefully accepted. We sit and chat for a while at Leah's bedside while she is watching some annoyingly screechy programme on CBeebies. She seems to be managing the chemo drugs incredibly well and hasn't really mentioned any side effects – so far, so good. I'm hoping I've overestimated the potential impact of the treatment and that she continues to deal with it all as well as she has for the last twenty-four hours. I guess only time will tell.

Our conversation then moves on to Phoebe and the fact that we haven't really spoken to her properly about the situation. In reality, we haven't really spoken to her about anything other than to quickly check in with her with a 'Hey, are you okay?' call via FaceTime. Such is the intensity of the situation and the volume of different discussions we have had with so many different people, Phoebe has definitely not had enough of our time. It hurts when I think about that. The impact that Leah's diagnosis is having on so many people is starting to become clear and I'm starting to feel guilty for failing as a parent with my other child. We both agree that we need to sit down and talk to her about everything sooner rather than later. I agree to do that tonight when I get home.

I collect Phoebe from Claire's parents' house on my way home from the hospital and we arrive back at our house at around 7pm. I want us to have dinner together, but she has already eaten with Claire's parents. Therefore, I just ask her to sit down at the kitchen table with me. It is now or never.

'Phoebe, I need to speak to you about Leah.' I sense this is a conversation she has been expecting, but not looking forward to. I feel exactly the same. She nervously sits down next to me. 'You know Leah has been in hospital a lot these last few weeks for tests? Well, the doctors have told us…' I feel a lump in my throat as I struggle with the words. 'The doctors have told us…' I pause again as my voice wobbles. 'The doctors have told us… that Leah… has… cancer.'

She stares back at me with her mouth slightly open

and I see the tears building in her eyes. She then bursts into tears, shaking her head in disbelief. I throw my arms around her and hug her tightly. Primarily as a show of affection and to comfort her, but also so she can't see the tears in my eyes. A minute or so later, while we are still holding each other, Phoebe asks me straight out, 'Is she going to die, Daddy?'

I probably should have prepared for that question before I started this conversation, but I didn't. In truth, I hadn't dare ask that question openly to anyone despite playing it out in my own head almost every night for the last two weeks. Now I had to provide an answer to a question I didn't dare to answer myself. Do I say 'no' and risk giving her false hope? Or do I say 'probably yes' and break her heart, but start to prepare her as early as possible for what looks to be the inevitable outcome. I decide that I can't say either and instead I go with what my heart cries out.

'I hope not, baby. I really hope not.'

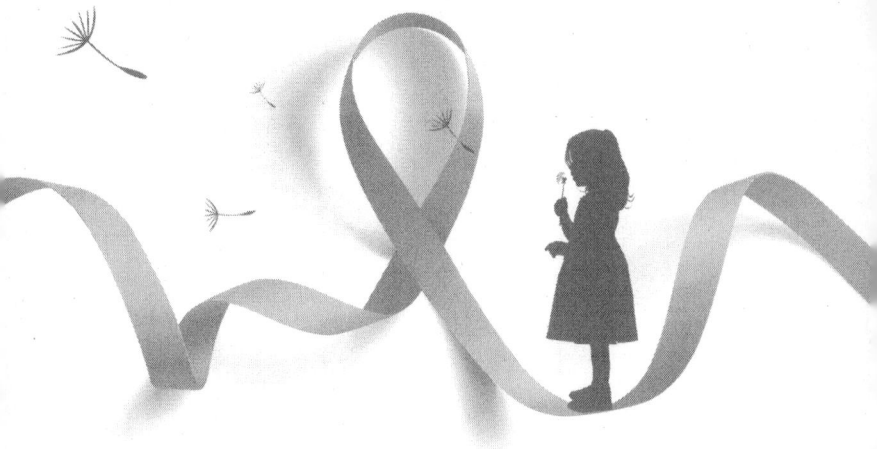

Big Sis

Phoebe is Leah's elder sister. The person who made Claire and I parents for the first time. Phoebe Marie Bennett. Her middle name from Claire's mum obviously, but also the name of my own nan, who Phoebe – and, in fact, Claire – sadly never got the chance to meet.

Phoebe is three years older than Leah, but was also a summer baby. This meant Claire and I spent ridiculous amounts of time worrying about how far behind the other kids in primary school she would be in terms of development. Given that some kids had almost a full year on her – and a year feels like an age during that time – it was a genuine concern. Then, all of a sudden, she hit high school and it just didn't seem to matter anymore!

I distinctly recall when we brought Leah home from the maternity ward to meet Phoebe for the first time. The way she looked at her in the baby carrier. She touched her tiny had and gave the biggest smile. A *real* dolly to play with! Three years between them in age was sufficient for Phoebe to safely assume the role of 'the older and more grown-up' sibling. But it wasn't too much to prevent them enjoying each other's company.

I have videos on my phone of them dressed as the princesses from *Frozen*, singing 'Let It Go' in full voice in the kitchen. Precious moments in time captured – and stored away for material for the embarrassing Dad speech at 18th birthdays or weddings. Of course, Phoebe got to be Elsa in the cooler dress. Being three years younger meant you were way down the pecking order when it came to the costume department!

As they got older, they inevitably started to fight more. Mainly because Leah started to rebel against the oppressive regime and refused to play the understudy all the time (aka Anna in terms of the *Frozen* performances).

You might expect two children born to the same two parents would be very similar in looks and character, but no. Hell, no! Leah has bucketloads of self-confidence and sass, whereas Phoebe is far more shy and timid. She is incredibly creative and has a great sense of humour, but carries round a bag full of anxiety a lot of the time. I suspect much of this emanates from the magnitude of the personal issues she has had to deal with during recent years. Seeing your grandmother struggling with cancer for a few years and then getting news of your sister's diagnosis would be a lot for anyone to deal with. However, it's easy to forget that Phoebe doesn't have the benefit of many, many years of calmer waters. In recent memory, she has only really sailed through the storm. That has to have an impact, right?

Whenever we go on an aeroplane for a holiday, Phoebe is white as a sheet and shaking with fear as she somehow convinces herself that the plane is going to plunge from the sky soon after take-off. I'm convinced this 'doom thinking' has its roots in our family situation. After all, the worst-case scenario has played out in front of her eyes many times in the early years of her life.

On one occasion, we were up in the house in Bute on holiday when Claire's dad offered to take us all out on his boat. We all jumped at the chance and so we set off for a day on the Clyde. The sun was shining and there were a number of smiling faces on board. Apart from one. Phoebe. She was sat below deck with her eyes closed.

'I'm so scared the boat will sink, Dad. The waves keep crashing against the sides and I hate it!'

'Phoebe, stop being so daft! The boat will not sink.'

We had a fantastic few hours out and stopped off in a bay at the foot of the island for a picnic. It was picture-perfect.

On the return journey, though, the weather started to change slightly and the wind started to strengthen. About half an hour into the sail home, the engine on the boat decided to give up and, all of a sudden, we found ourselves floating about thirty metres off the coast of the island. To make matters worse, the auxiliary engine was also refusing to fire up and the wind was starting to push the boat towards the rocky edge of the river!

To cut a very long and dramatic story short, the

boat ended up being smashed against the rocks and was completely destroyed. Thankfully, everyone managed to disembark before that happened, but, for Phoebe, it was almost a complete validation of her fear. The worst obviously *does* always happen to her.

Leah's diagnosis has undoubtedly been life-changing for Leah. It certainly has been for Claire and I. It's probably easy to overlook how life-changing it's also been for Phoebe. Psychologically, it has potentially done more invisible damage to her than many of us realise.

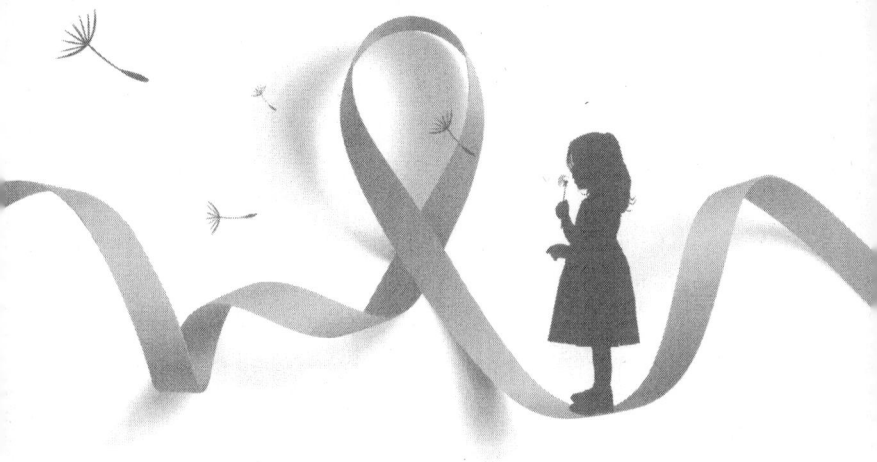

The Marathon

Just after breakfast, I repack my overnight bag and head back into the hospital with Phoebe. She has asked if she can go in to see Leah after our conversation last night. When we arrive on the ward, I sense Phoebe is a little nervous about seeing her sister, probably because she doesn't know fully what to expect. We head into the bay to see Claire sat next to Leah's bed. Phoebe runs up to her and gives her a big hug before turning her attention to Leah. She already seems less nervous – I'm guessing because she can see Leah is sat up in bed and talking, even though she looks a little pale and tired.

Claire tells me that Leah struggled a little overnight as the first signs of the side effects from the chemo drugs appeared. She vomited a few times in the early hours of the morning. She also didn't eat anything for breakfast.

The nurses have connected a bottle of what looks like thick beige milk to a small pump on the drip stand next to her bed and it is being given to her via the PEG tube in her stomach. The bottle is half empty so I assume she has tolerated that this morning.

Claire looks tired and haunted by the whole experience, which is probably exactly how I would describe my own look if I could see it. Leah, although she is sat up talking to Phoebe, looks weak and ill. None of us are shaping up particularly well already and we've only just started on this long journey.

Sunday 24th February 2019

We reached the end of the first round of Leah's chemotherapy today. She was not sick overnight and she slept a lot, so she seems a tiny bit better this morning, although she is definitely still not herself and is really pale and in a constant degree of discomfort.

Just before midday, the nurses come to disconnect Leah from the drip stand. Before they do, they carry out the normal nursing observations that they do every couple of hours and check her blood pressure, her oxygen saturation levels and her temperature. Claire and I have started to pack up all our belongings in bags ready to go home. I can't wait to get us all home and be reunited as a family of four again. The nurse looking after Leah puts the digital thermometer into Leah's left ear and it bleeps to confirm a reading has been taken. 38.2°C flashes up on the monitor next to the bed.

'Oh, you're a bit warm, aren't you, Leah?' says the nurse. 'I'll have to speak to the doctor on duty and see what she wants us to do.' This does not sound promising.

Five minutes later, Mary, one of the more experienced nurses in the team, comes over to Leah's bed to explain the situation. Essentially, chemotherapy treatment disrupts the process that the bone marrow uses to create blood cells. Blood cells include some white cells called neutrophils, which are the key weapon in fighting infection around the body. Therefore, if someone undergoing chemotherapy contracts an infection and they have low levels of neutrophils to fight it, it can be extremely dangerous and potentially fatal to them. A raised temperature is one of the early warning signs of infection and therefore they cannot allow Leah to go home until they are comfortable that she is free from infection.

We were previously advised of the need to regularly monitor her temperature whenever she is at home in between treatments. We were also advised to bring her into the hospital as quickly as possible if her temperature is 38°C or above. It doesn't look like that particular piece of advice is going to be relevant right now, as it's unlikely she is coming home any time soon.

Half an hour later and that situation is confirmed by one of the doctors. Leah is hooked back up to a pump on the drip stand and a two-day course of antibiotics is commenced. Leah is devastated. She was desperate to go home. We are devastated, too. We were desperate to take her home. Claire and I unpack the bags.

Monday 25th February 2019

Despite the situation, I'm trying really hard to accept that we are in this for the long haul now and that we just need to make the best of a bad situation. We need to understand what is happening to our daughter and also understand the role we have to play in terms of giving her every chance to overcome this.

I bump into the same oncology registrar on the ward that we met on the 11th February. He smiles and asks how we are getting on. I tell him we are as fine as we can be and that we are slowly starting to get our heads around the situation.

He replies, 'We see that a lot with our families. After they get over the initial shock, they realise that they are just part of a huge team running a marathon.' I guess he's right, but I'd much rather have to run a marathon (or twenty).

Today, though, we are scheduled to meet Kelly, one of the community nurses employed by a company called Abbot, who supply the bottled feed (aka beige milk) and pumps to the hospital. Kelly is supposed to be coming to our house to train us up to administer the nutritional feed at home when Leah is out of hospital. Because Leah is now staying in, she comes to the ward and delivers the training at Leah's bedside. I suppose this is just one of our first tasks as part of the 'team running the marathon'.

Later in the afternoon, we are asked to take Leah down to the radiology department again – this time for a bone scan. I haven't fully absorbed all the info from the meeting with Prof. Pilling, but my crude understanding of its purpose is to look at whether the cancer in Leah's spine is also visible in any of the other bones in her body. I agree to take Leah down while Claire returns home to repack the overnight bags.

We arrive in the radiology department and a lovely, cheerful lady called Emma greets us and takes us into a small room, where Leah is injected with some sort of dye. Emma explains that it is actually a radioactive substance[10] that effectively 'sticks to the bones' and shows up any areas of concern. The 'dye' takes a couple of hours to get round the body, so we go back up the ward and return to the gamma camera suite in radiology later that afternoon.

When we return, Emma again greets us and chats to Leah before showing us into the scanning room. Leah gets up onto the scanning table and a large square panel is lowered over her until it stops quite close to her face. She looks a little like she is lying in a huge toastie maker. The table then slowly starts to pull her so that her whole body will eventually pass underneath the 'Breville'.

I am sat a couple of metres away, staring at the monitor above the scanner, which is (possibly inadvertently) facing where I am sat. As Leah's upper body passes through the toaster, the monitor displays the output from the scanner. I can make out Leah's body shape, and her skeleton is twinkling like an elaborate constellation in the night sky. It is fascinatingly beautiful.

As she passes further under the scanner, a large bright white blob starts to appear on the screen. It is the tumour. Illuminated again in front of my eyes. Glistening and

10 Great – more awful poison being pushed into her body!

almost taunting me. It feels like it takes forever to disappear from the view again. Leah's lower abdomen then starts to pass under the scanner and, to my utter horror, another bright white blob starts to become visible at the bottom of the screen.

Oh God, no! I'm thinking. *Please, no!* But it is there, shining brightly back at me. There is only one explanation here surely. She must have another tumour further down. I can feel the life leaving my body and I'm trying my best to remain composed. How am I going to break this news to Claire? I don't know what it is, so I can't break the news to her. I wouldn't be able to answer her questions. I'll need to wait until we see Prof. Pilling tomorrow and he can break the news to us together. I have no idea how I'm going to sit on this for twenty-four hours. Already I'm beyond stressed and agitated.

The bleakest of situations has just hit yet another new low.

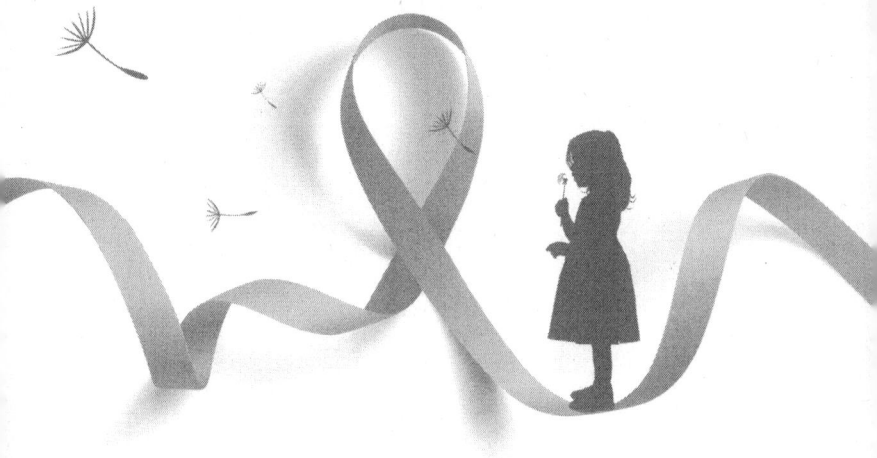

The Oncology Family

I distinctly remember one of the nurses on the oncology ward saying to me quite early on that we should take time to speak to other parents and families on the ward. She said we would get a lot of helpful advice from that source – arguably more helpful than some of the advice from the clinical teams.

A couple of weeks after Leah's initial diagnosis, I wander into the parents' kitchen on the ward to make myself a (strong) coffee. When I open the door, there is a guy with shoulder-length auburn hair standing next to the kettle making himself a drink. He turns round and shoots me a smile, which I return. He introduces himself as Tom and says, 'Hi!' He has a really friendly demeanour and seems to be full of energy[11].

---

11   In fairness, I think a sloth holding a flat car battery would probably be perceived as being 'full of energy' compared to me right now.

For the next fifteen minutes, Tom and I talk. He clearly recognised me as a 'newbie' on the ward as I was probably still displaying that 'rabbit in the headlights' look, and he had obviously been plodding along this painful path a little longer than I had.

He is happy to give me a few hints and tips about life on 3B and I am grateful to receive them:

1. 'Get yourselves a parking pass, otherwise you'll be paying a fortune for car parking every day.' (*Erm, too late, but thanks.*)
2. 'There are some charities who will cook a hot meal for you for free once a month if you are stuck in the hospital and struggling.'
3. 'Make sure you write your name on your milk, otherwise they throw it out when they clean the fridge every few days.'

It turns out that Tom and his partner, Suzie, have been on the oncology roller coaster with their son, Jaxon, for almost nine months, which I guess is why he knows so much. Jaxon hasn't really responded to any chemotherapy treatment to date so they are exploring the options that might be available to him. Tom has been juggling work down south and overseas with spending time in the hospital as often as he can. Suzie, on the other hand, has spent the last nine months with Jaxon in room four – one of the side rooms on the ward. Day in, day out, just cooped up in that small room. Like Tom Hanks in the film, *The Terminal*.

Tom describes how the experience has given him the opportunity to spend real quality time with his son and his partner. He'd shared some really special moments over the last nine months with them, which he may not ordinarily have had the chance to do. I find it quite astonishing that he is able to find some positives from the complete shit-show that his life has become. It really makes me think. I thank Tom for his help and advice and say that I hope they will find an answer to help Jaxon. Tom thanks me and wanders back to room four. As he slides the door open, I get a glimpse inside the room. Suzie is sat there cradling Jaxon. Their belongings are scattered around the room. Everything important to them is encapsulated in a single tiny space.

Over the course of the next few weeks and months, Claire and I would find out more and more about this world we were now part of. We even found ourselves being able to identify the newbies ourselves and passing on advice to others. We became part of the oncology family. A group of people who truly understand how this all feels. They've shared the hope and the fears. They've shared the tears and the lack of sleep. They've worked out where to get the best cup of coffee at 8am on a Saturday morning.

These are people we need and who need us, too. We're all in this together.

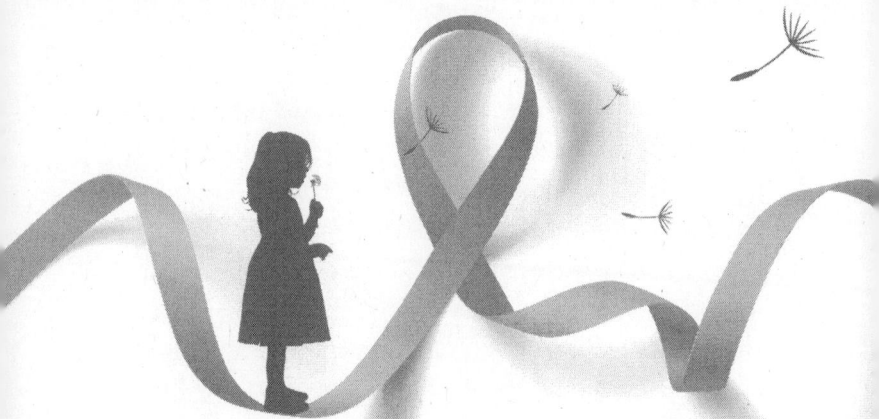

On the Pillow

Tuesday 26th February 2019

Claire stayed in the hospital last night with Leah and I stayed at home with Phoebe, who is getting more and more clingy by the day. She refused to sleep in her own bed last night, so I let her get in with me so that she wasn't on her own. That seemed to help a little. Well, it seemed to help Phoebe. I, on the other hand, hardly slept a wink all night. I had the image of those two big white blobs on the screen going through my head. I have to keep telling myself to stop overthinking because I don't know what it means until I've had the chance to speak to Prof. Pilling later today. I'm so worried, though, and I feel like I'm hiding all this from Claire, but what do I gain from telling her?

I drop Phoebe off at school and set off back to the hospital. I still can't think of anything other than that scan and what I'm convinced I'm about to be hit with by Prof. Pilling.

I arrive on the ward again and find Leah's bed empty and Claire nowhere to be seen. I ask one of the nurses if they know where they are and I get directed to the classroom at the top of the ward. I pop my head around the door and, true enough, there is Leah sat in a wheelchair, playing on some drums with a big smile on her face. Immediately, it makes me smile and, for a split second, all my worries disappear. Jo, the classroom teacher, is encouraging Leah to bash the drums and make as much noise as she can. Leah duly responds and does her best impression of 'Animal' from the Muppets. It is amazing to watch her carefree and having fun, just like a six-year-old child should be.

Just after lunch, Prof. Pilling comes over to Leah's bed and asks Claire and I to follow him into one of the consulting rooms for a quick chat. I gulp hard. I know what is coming. Claire is oblivious to the bombshell that is about to drop and I feel guilty about that. I feel sick.

We follow him into the room and sit down opposite a small desk in the corner. 'Okay, so Leah had a bone scan yesterday,' Prof. Pilling starts. I am almost adopting the brace position. I can't look him in the eye and I'm just waiting for the words 'I'm really sorry but…' to come out of his mouth. 'I've had a quick look at the scan this morning,' he continues. Here it comes. I close my eyes. Three, two, one and…

'The scan looks okay. There is no evidence of further spread of the disease in any other bones in her body, which is good news.'

I let out the biggest breath and almost immediately the tension leaves my body. I was wrong. I was completely wrong! Thankfully, I was so bloody wrong. I've never been more pleased to be wrong about anything in my life!

In hindsight, I can only assume that the other 'white blob' I saw on the scan was just her bladder and the dye must have just been collecting in there. They really need to stop letting parents see the screens when the scans are in progress – especially idiotic, overthinking parents like me!

Wednesday 27th February 2019

Leah's temperature remains higher than it should be and the medical team are still trying to work out what is causing it. This means that there is still no sign of her being allowed home any time soon.

Later in the day, Leah is sat up in bed, watching TV, but she is really struggling with pain and discomfort in her lower back. In truth, she has been complaining about this for a number of days and it seems to be gradually getting worse. To the point where she is now struggling to cope with it and it is making her upset. The team on 3B put a call out to the urology team to come and review Leah. A couple of hours later, one of the senior urology registrars appears to see Leah and to talk to Claire and I.

He tells us that the urology team are aware of Leah through the recent oncology MDT meetings. He explains that the size and location of the tumour in Leah's abdomen is causing a problem with regards to the drainage of her kidneys, particularly her right one, and as a result they are starting to swell. This is highly likely to be the source of her pain.

The urology team have adopted a 'watch and wait' stance with regards to Leah's kidneys, hoping – I think – that the chemo treatment might shrink the tumour effectively and relieve some pressure on her other organs. However, she is struggling with the pain so much that we're not happy that 'watch and wait' is the right answer. The registrar notes our concerns and tells us that he will go and discuss the situation with one of the consultants and come back to us.

An hour later, he returns along with one of the urology consultants, a friendly lady with wispy grey hair called Miss McAndrew. Miss McAndrew then proceeds to explain that she has agreed that they need to act sooner than they had intended in order to help Leah. She informs us that Leah is to return to theatre tomorrow to have a stent inserted into each of her urethras in order to help drain her kidneys. This is yet another blow and Leah is really upset to hear it. However, based upon the fact that she is now visibly struggling with the pain, it is clear that something needs to be done urgently.

Claire covers the night shift and messages me to say that Leah's pain is getting worse and worse as the night draws on. At one point in the early hours, she was lying awake, screaming in agony. By all accounts, it was another harrowing experience for everyone involved. At another point during the night, the on-call anaesthetist needed to be summoned to put Leah on strong pain medication delivered via a special infusion pump. Claire told me that this seemed to help and, at around 3am, she eventually fell asleep.

Thursday 28th February 2019

Having been told about the difficulties of last night, I drop Phoebe at school and go directly to Alder Hey to be with Claire and Leah. We know that Leah is going to theatre today, but we just hope it will be earlier rather than later given her struggles. Leah is in acute pain and has barely slept. She is also aware of the plan to take her back to theatre today and she is obviously frightened about it.

She seemed to cope well with the trip to theatre the last time she went, so we are assuming that she will be okay going back this time – an assumption that we couldn't have got more wrong in hindsight.

At around 10am, two of the theatre porters arrive with an empty trolley to collect her. She spots them enter the bay and immediately screams and lashes out.

'I'm not going, Mummy! I'm not doing it! I'm really scared!' she shouts. It is really upsetting for all of us. The reality of the situation is that we have no choice here. She could end up with kidney failure quite quickly if we don't do something about this, yet she is too young and far too scared to comprehend this. Despite the porter's best efforts to calm her down with a few of their tried-and-tested jokes and tricks, she eventually only agrees to come down if I carry her. So that's what I do.

When we get down to the anaesthetic room, Leah becomes extremely distressed again. The room is again full of a number of strange faces. Her eyes dart around the room and, as quick as a flash, she jumps off the trolley and runs into the corner of the room away from everyone. She is refusing to allow the anaesthetist access to her central line. Craftily, she has worked out that they can't put her to sleep without using the central line, so she has managed to take control of the situation[12]. Claire and I know how important it is that she has these stents inserted and also know that she has a defined slot on the emergency theatre list, so we are adamant that she has to go inside as quickly as possible or risk losing the slot altogether.

After around twenty minutes of trying to convince Leah to co-operate, the suggestion is made to perhaps try and sedate her back in the surgical admissions lounge and then try again when the sedative has kicked in. Claire and I agree, so we lead Leah out of the room and back to the admissions lounge where we are shown into one of the side rooms and one of the theatre nurses come in to 'check Leah's lines'[13]. After around ten minutes, Leah has calmed right down and is now lying on Claire's knee looking decidedly sleepy. We opt to try again. I scoop her up from Claire's lap and we make our way back to the anaesthetic room for attempt number two.

We walk down the corridor and turn the corner to where the doors to the anaesthetic room are. As soon as it dawns on Leah where we are heading, BANG, she sits bolt upright

---

12 With the benefit of hindsight, I am extremely proud of her intuition and determination in this situation. At the time, I could have murdered her!

13 I.e. administer the sedative.

and turns into the child from *The Exorcist* again, screaming and crying (and that's just me). I decide that we have to take a much more direct approach or risk missing the opportunity to help her. I place her on the trolley and then have to physically restrain her arms and shoulders to allow the anaesthetist to access her central line. I look at her and her face is bright red, her eyes streaming with tears. She screams in my face, '*Daddy, help me!*' I will never, ever forget that moment for as long as I live. I glare at the anaesthetist; my eyes saying, 'Bloody get on with it!' He takes the hint and leans to connect the syringe of anaesthetic medicine to her line.

At that point, Leah kicks his hand and the milky white liquid squirts all over his theatre scrubs and splashes over Leah's face. I didn't think it was possible for her to hit a higher level of distress, but at that point she hit DEFCON one. The anaesthetist quickly connects the syringe and pushes in the drugs. Leah goes floppy in my grip and it is done. Calmness descends on the room and there is a collective sigh. Forty-five minutes after we started trying, she is finally asleep and ready to go into the theatre. Claire and I kiss her on the forehead and leave the room. Outside, the tension and emotion bursts from us both and we break down in tears, shaking.

We go to meet Leah in recovery an hour later. She refuses to say a word to either of us (again).

Friday 1st March 2019

The insertion of the stents seems to have been a big success and Leah wakes up this morning free from the pain and discomfort in her back that she has been experiencing over recent days. The nursing observations are all showing normal temperature levels and no areas of concern. As a result, the medical teams have confirmed that she can possibly go home tomorrow, as long as she remains stable and comfortable for the remainder of the day.

She is absolutely shattered after going ten rounds with her parents and half the theatre staff yesterday, so she sleeps on and off for most of the day. That evening, I help her to wash her body in the bathroom and she puts on some fresh pyjamas. She gets back into her bed and I raise her up using the bed controls, so that I can brush her hair. I look down at the brush and there are large clumps of hair stuck in the bristles. There is more on her pillow and around the bed. I quickly clean it up so she doesn't notice.

But I notice. And it really hurts.

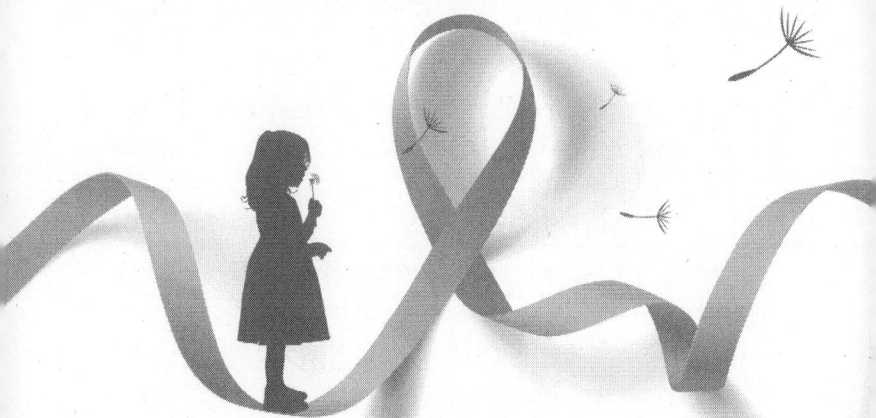

She's Electric

Saturday 2nd March 2019

Ten days after Leah was admitted to Alder Hey to commence her first three-day chemotherapy treatment, she is finally allowed to come home. Claire and Phoebe travel into the hospital to help us pack up all of our things and, just after lunch, the ward team hand us some discharge paperwork and a huge bag of anti-sickness and pain medication. One of the senior nurses, Marianne, comes in to speak to Claire and I. She is here to answer any questions we have and make sure we are confident to manage Leah's condition at home over the coming days. At eight minutes past two in the afternoon, we finally walk off the ward. Together. The relief is almost tangible.

We get to the car park and load up both Claire's boot and my boot full of bags of clothes, food, tablet computers, toilet bags, colouring books and various bits of Play-Doh. Phoebe decides that she wants to come home in my car and so does Leah, so Claire sets off separately and the girls and I travel home along the M62 in my car.

On the way, 'She's Electric' by Oasis comes on the radio. It is a song that Leah and I have sung together a few times[14]. The three of us sing it together at full belt with big smiles on our faces as we fly down the motorway. I can't describe how special the moment feels. For the first time in what feels like forever, I can feel the wind on my face (quite literally as I've got the windows open in the car).

Leah sleeps in our bed tonight and Claire and I both wrap our arms around her and fall asleep. I almost didn't want to sleep because I didn't want to forget how good today felt, but my exhausted body and mind had other plans and I'm soon out for the count.

Sunday 3rd March 2019

At home, we are required to replicate the frequency and doses of the various medicines that Leah was receiving in the hospital throughout the day. Six-hourly anti-sickness medication and regular temperature checks is going to become our daily rhythm, I suspect. Leah's temperature has remained stable all day, thankfully, so we've managed a full day at home together.

---

14 In my unashamed attempts to teach her 'proper' music before the marketing hypnotists of the world of pop music try to brainwash her.

Just before lunchtime, we have a visit from one of the Alder Hey oncology outreach nurses, who comes to take a small sample of Leah's blood and administer something called GCSF. The GCSF helps the bone marrow to produce more white blood cells to help her fight any infection that might threaten her safety[15]. The outreach team will come to our home every day when Leah is out of hospital to give her the GCSF and check the impact it is having on her blood count. It is quite incredible how much we have all learned about this hidden world in such a short space of time. None of it is through choice, though.

Later in the afternoon, I reluctantly make the phone call to cancel our planned holiday to Italy in the summer. We had only booked it a matter of weeks ago. At least for the few weeks leading up to that fateful day on the 6th of February, we were all excited and had something to look forward to. I have no idea whether we would ever get to Italy now and, if we did, would we get there as a family of four?

I desperately fight to hold it together as I explain the situation to the representative from the travel company over the phone. He listens to me for about five minutes before robotically apologising for the fact that we have received the bad news. He then proceeds to read the terms and conditions of the booking directly from a script in a monotone voice. He finishes with the delightful news that our £600 deposit is, in fact, non-refundable and will

---

15 GCSF stands for Granulocyte Colony-Stimulating Factor.
    Remember bone marrow = white blood cells = infection fighting
    = safer from harm.

therefore not be returned to us. I don't have the energy to argue with him. To be honest, everything about the last few weeks has felt like the plagues of Egypt are slowly being unleashed on us, so, on that basis, being told we've lost £600 feels relatively insignificant.

Monday 4th March 2019

I've been woken really early this morning by the alarm on Leah's feed pump. There is a blockage somewhere in the tube going from the pump to her PEG tube and the milk is therefore unable to pass through. Leah is still sleeping in our bed, which isn't really designed for three people and she's rolled onto the tube. I gently roll her off the tube, reset the pump and settle back down to sleep. This happens at least two more times in the night before the pump finally alarms to signify that the milk carton is empty and it has all been pumped into Leah's stomach.

I finally wake after another terrible night's sleep to see a lot more hair on the pillow around Leah's head. We are picking up fistfuls of hair on a daily basis and her scalp is visibly thinning. A little girl's pride and joy should be her beautiful hair and this awful disease is even stealing that from her. Stealing her dignity.

To cheer the girls up and act as a slight distraction to the horrors of daily life, Claire and I have agreed to buy them both a new pet. Later that afternoon, we trek down to the local pet shop. They look at the rabbits, rats, chinchillas and even snakes, but eventually, with perhaps a little parental persuasion, settle on hamsters. They missed a trick really. They could have probably asked for a herd of glittery unicorns and we would have found them and bought them, so I feel two hamsters with cages and a huge bag of sawdust is definitely a bullet dodged.

Phoebe picks a tan-and-white one and Leah chooses a slightly smaller, scruffy-looking black-and-white one. They are only ten pounds each, but I can't help feeling that Leah's doesn't look the healthiest rodent on planet Earth. Putting it in a slightly different way, I'll be keeping the receipt!

Leah proudly names her hamster 'Harry' after her favourite book character, a certain Mr Potter, so Phoebe falls in line and calls hers 'Ginny'. And yes, we did confirm Harry was a boy and Ginny a girl, hence two very separate cages.

Tuesday 5th March 2019

My mum has a friend from work called Lisa who used to be a hairdresser in a former life. Lisa has kindly offered to come round to cut Leah's hair short, on the basis that it might just make it slightly less upsetting for her when it finally all falls out.

It is both beautiful and heartbreaking to watch in equal measure. Beautiful because Lisa is desperately trying to show her support and help Leah and our family, in the tiniest way. But it is utterly heartbreaking as Lisa's hairbrush is pulling more and more hair out. She is essentially just cutting a small amount off a few strands of hair and brushing the hair that remains across her scalp to cover it as best she can. Leah seems happy with the job

Lisa has done. Lisa looks like she is fighting back tears with every stroke of the hairbrush. Claire and I are just a complete mess.

Wednesday 6th March 2019

A thankfully uneventful day scheduled for today. Only the (now usual) home visit from the oncology outreach team needs to be accommodated. Today's member of the team is Becky. She is a short lady with dark hair and a round face. Immediately, it feels like there is something different about Becky. In fairness, all of the staff we've met from Alder Hey over the past few whirlwind weeks have been pretty incredible and really caring, but Becky is just on a level above. It is the first time we've met her and she already feels like part of our family. She just seems desperate to help us out in any way she can.

She comes to take a small sample of blood from Leah's central line and then goes on her way (after a quick brew and a small piece of chocolate cake). Off to walk into the home of another local family whose lives have been torn apart by this disease, no doubt.

Later that afternoon, Becky calls us to tell us that Leah's bloods are good[16] and therefore she is okay to commence round two of chemotherapy the following day as planned. I'm not really sure whether that is something to be happy about or not? Another brew and another slice of chocolate cake help me decide it probably is, just.

---

16 Bloods are good = levels of red cells, platelets and, most importantly, white cells are at an acceptably safe level.

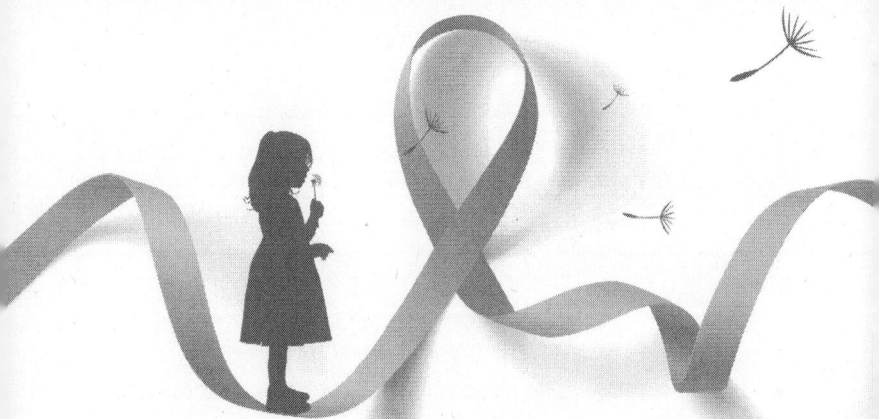

Bright Red Bag

Thursday 7th March 2019

Round two of chemo starts today. For the next six – yes, *six* days – Leah will be reattached to the pumps on the drip stand as she receives the IE element of the VDC-IE treatment. We arrive on the ward at 9am and she's been allocated a bed in the four-bedded bay again. I'm already regretting not packing my thermals for sleeping in sub-arctic temperatures next to the window. She settles onto the bed and, after a short review by one of the advanced nurse practitioners (ANPs), she is given the green light to proceed with the treatment.

About half an hour later, two of the nurses come over to her bed. They are both covered head to toe in PPE[17]. One is

---

17 Personal Protective Equipment (apron, gloves, face masks etc.).
    It did exist before coronavirus made it fashionable.

carrying a large grey tray containing syringes, tubes, wipes and various packages – aka drug paraphernalia. The other nurse is struggling to carry two large bags of fluids. One of the bags has a shiny, bright red plastic jacket around it and the other appears to be a huge bag of water, which wouldn't look out of place hanging from a fairground stall with a goldfish swimming in it[18].

I watch the nurses check that the details on the bags match the details on Leah's hospital wristbands, then they start to hook the bags to the pumps on the drip stands. I look closely at the writing on the red bag. It has large visible hazardous crosses drawn on it and the words 'WARNING: CONTAINS CYTOTOXIC MATERIALS' written across the front. The nurses advise us to wear the same PPE as them whenever helping Leah to the toilet while she is having this treatment.

What the hell is this fucking shit they are putting into my little girl?! Cytotoxic. So poisonous that I need to wear PPE to protect me when helping her to the toilet. It will make her sick and her hair fall out and her mouth ulcerate and it will probably ruin her kidneys. Yet we have no idea whether this will actually help her to survive this nightmare[19]. *What. The. Fuck?*

I pause to reflect on this intensely painful juxtaposition.

---

18 It turns out that these bags of water are actually saline solution used to help keep the body hydrated during the treatment, in order to lessen the potential impact of any side effects.

19 Ifosfamide, like cyclophosphamide, another of the drugs used to treat Leah, is actually created as a derivative of the chemical weapon mustard gas used in World War I. This might help to give you a sense of just how damaging this stuff is.

Every fabric of my being is screaming out for them to stop feeding this poison into my little girl. But, deep down, I know that she probably had no chance of survival without it. So, I have no choice but to sit there and watch them do it. And smile. And thank the staff. 'Thank you for poisoning my daughter.'

How on earth did we end up here?

Friday 8th March 2019

Leah has woken up in a foul mood today after a bad night's sleep. The pumps on the drip stand seemed to beep every ten minutes for one reason or another during the night and she needed multiple trips to the toilet. She's already vomited into a bowl twice between 7:30am and 10am.

After lunchtime, we have a visit from the local representative from a charity called CLIC Sargent[20]. The CLIC Sargent rep for Alder Hey is a man called Mike. He is probably in his mid to late thirties, dressed in a T-shirt and jeans, with a vivid purple lanyard around his neck.

He comes and sits down next to Leah's bed and talks to Claire and I. He wants to know about Leah, about our family situation and, most importantly, he wants to know how he can help us. He has a really friendly manner and he quickly starts to get Leah to talk, which is way more than I've managed this morning, so I like him already.

Leah spots Mike's surname on the ID badge attached to his lanyard – Mike Nugent.

'Is your name Nugget?' she asks him.

---

20   CLIC Sargent has since rebranded as Young Lives vs Cancer.

He laughs loudly. 'That was my nickname at school – how did you know?' Mike replies. 'Just because it's you, I'll let you call me Nugget, but don't tell anyone else, okay?'

'Okay,' says Leah, with a smile.

'How would you like to design your own pair of trainers, Miss Leah?' Mike asks her.

Leah's eyes light up and she gives him a double thumbs up.

'Well, next time I come and see you, I'll bring the form for you to fill in and you can do just that.' Mike has already helped us just by getting Leah to smile today. Sometimes it's the simple things. Although I do suspect he might regret letting Leah call him Nugget.

I spend some time going through my phone today, reading and trying to respond to a near constant stream of messages that I've received over the last week or so. Messages from people close to me and messages from people further afield, but all with the same tone. Horrified to hear what's happened and desperate to help in any way. Unless any of them have an instant cure for cancer, then I'm not sure what more I can ask from them. However, the sheer volume of messages is enough to reinforce the fact that we have an army of support behind us already and that is something I'm drawing a degree of strength from.

Just before I leave the hospital for the evening for Claire to take over, Marie and Peter come to visit. Peter is pushing Marie in a wheelchair. This rocks me slightly as it is the first time I've seen Marie so unwell that she is unable to walk by herself. She is pale and looks tired. Seeing her like this is a quick reminder of the wider challenges facing our family right now. Despite her own obvious struggles, she is here to see her granddaughter and show her support for her daughter. She is demonstrating the grit and determination that we will all need to show in the weeks, months, years (?) ahead. She is one amazing lady.

Saturday 9th March 2019

Claire did the overnight stay at the hospital last night and I stayed at home with Phoebe. She asked to sleep on Claire's side of our bed instead of in her own. Of course I agreed. In fact, I really loved being close to her. She needed to know I was there for her and I just needed a cuddle.

Later in the morning, Phoebe and I set off to the hospital. I call Claire on the way in and she tells me that she's had another difficult night. Leah was so exhausted from constantly broken sleep that it got to the point where she shuffled over to the bathroom in the early hours of the morning and sat on the toilet in floods of tears, saying, 'I can't do this anymore, Mummy. I hate my life.'

Hearing that really upsets me, so I can only imagine how tough it would have been for Claire. Not only do we have to find ways to keep each other going, we also have to find ways to keep Leah's spirits up. However, it sounds like Claire, thinking on her feet, has already solved that particular problem. She has promised Leah that we will throw the biggest party when her treatment ends and she can invite anyone she wants. They then spent half an hour discussing who they would invite to the party. It seems that it has worked a treat in picking Leah back up.

The age-old art of distraction works again as the primary weapon in any parent's arsenal! I'm just so terrified that we might never get the chance to fulfil this promise.

Sunday 10th March 2019

I did the night shift last night and it was particularly tough. Leah woke me up every two hours (almost on the dot) to help her go to the toilet. Each time, I have to unplug the three pumps from the wall, wrap the power leads around the drip stand, press the mute button on each of them to stop them beeping hysterically (because the power has been cut), help Leah down from the bed and across the bay to the bathroom, wheeling the drip stand in close proximity behind her. It is exhausting for both of us.

She is struggling, but I know she won't give up and she makes me so proud. There was one trip to the bathroom during the night where she wobbled and started the 'I can't do this, Daddy' conversation, but I pulled out the party card and it worked a treat. My wife is a genius! Cunning, but a genius!

Monday 11th March 2019

The impact of the last month of broken and minimal sleep is really starting to hit Claire and I now. Others close to us have clearly noticed it, too, as Claire's sister, Amy, has agreed to cover the night shift for us tonight. I'm a little nervous about this, to be honest. I'm only just starting to get my head around all the things I need to do to look after her while she's in hospital myself, so I don't want to overburden Amy with the responsibility. However, she is a sensible woman, so I don't doubt that she'll pick it up. Besides, we're completely knackered, so we probably don't have much choice.

Claire has agreed to stay in the hospital with Leah today and do the handover to Amy later, so that I can go home and start work on Leah's new bedroom. This is something Claire and I have been discussing for a few weeks now. Leah sleeping in our room means that none of us really get to sleep properly while we are at home. That's not great for any of us. Therefore, I'm off to Ikea to buy a new single bed to put up in our spare bedroom. The idea is that we convert it into a kind of hospital room at home, so that one of us can sleep in with Leah while the other gets some much-needed rest.

I leave Ikea over £500 lighter and somehow manage to cram the whole flat-packed lot of it into the back of Claire's Vauxhall Mokka, successfully avoiding the £45 delivery fee. I'm turning more and more into my father every day.

Once at home, I adopt the typical masculine approach of tearing open the boxes and trying to work out how to put it all together with only fleeting glances at the instructions. After around two hours and several assemblies and dis-assemblies later, I follow the instructions to the letter and, hey presto, we have a new bed set up. I also screw a small whiteboard to the wall, so that we can scribble down when she needs all her medicines during the day.

It makes me feel so much better once this is all

complete, as it feels like we are more prepared. At the same time, it makes me feel really upset as it is yet another example of just how far from 'normal' our lives have now become. I'm also a little pissed off that I've lost some 'dad points' for resorting to reading the Ikea instructions, if I'm totally honest.

Tuesday 12th March 2019

Both Claire and I stayed at home last night and we slept in the same bed together, without one of our daughters, for the first time since the 4th of February. Neither of us is struggling to sleep at the moment. I think this is a combination of general emotional exhaustion and the fact that life has settled more into a routine. It may only have been one night we got together, but it was so important to be able to talk freely and remind each other that we had each other's backs.

I'm back on hospital duty tonight, so I head off to Alder Hey at lunchtime to take over from Amy. When I get there, both Leah and Amy are laughing together and look like they've been okay. Immediately seeing them like this makes me feel at ease. Leah is not happy that Amy is going home and handing back over to me. I don't take it personally; she is bored of me and I don't blame her! She's obviously had fun with Auntie Amy last night, playing games and watching films. Having boring, grumpy Dad back in the room is definitely a downgrade for her. I thank Amy and she looks pleased to have been able to help us before she heads off home. She has left Leah with a spare iPhone she has managed to get hold of from somewhere. A bored Leah and instant access to FaceTime on an iPhone preloaded with Amy's number feels like a schoolboy error to me, but best of luck to her!

Later in the afternoon, Leah gets invited into the classroom on the ward by Jo the ward teacher. She's going to take part in a session drawing cartoons with members of a company called Comic Youth. Leah draws a cartoon of Harry the hamster visiting a hospital for hamsters and the Comic Youth team help fuel her imagination and make her smile. It is moments like these when Leah is transported a million miles away from the reality of life on chemotherapy. Watching her smile and get involved is just magical. Look out for the adventures of Harry the hamster as the sequel to this book.

Wednesday 13th March 2019

Today is the final day of chemo round two. This cycle of six days has been really hard work for us all. It is exhausting and we are all desperate to get home.

After the usual daily ward round, where the consultant on duty confirms they are happy for Leah to leave hospital later today, thankfully, we have a visit from one of the occupational therapy (OT) team.

The other major issue with Leah's health at the moment relates to her mobility. She is unable to sit upright for more than a few minutes due to the pressure of the tumour on her lower back and the damage the cancer is doing to the bottom of her spine. It is tough to see my little girl like this.

A girl who was playing football, skiing and swimming just a couple of months ago now needing specialist equipment to get round. However, she needs to be able to get out of the house and enjoy her life away from the hospital as much as possible, so I know it's for the best.

The OT team come to assess Leah and agree to source us a specialist armchair for her to sit in at home, as well as a specialist mobility buggy to allow us to get her out of the house. Both the buggy and the armchair will allow her to recline and reduce the pressure on her back so I feel positive that they will make a difference for her. The equipment is expected to be delivered to our home in the next few days.

At around 4:30pm, we are given a huge bag of medicines and a discharge letter from the ward staff, and we pack our multiple bags and leave Ward 3B after six long days. She's definitely coming home this time.

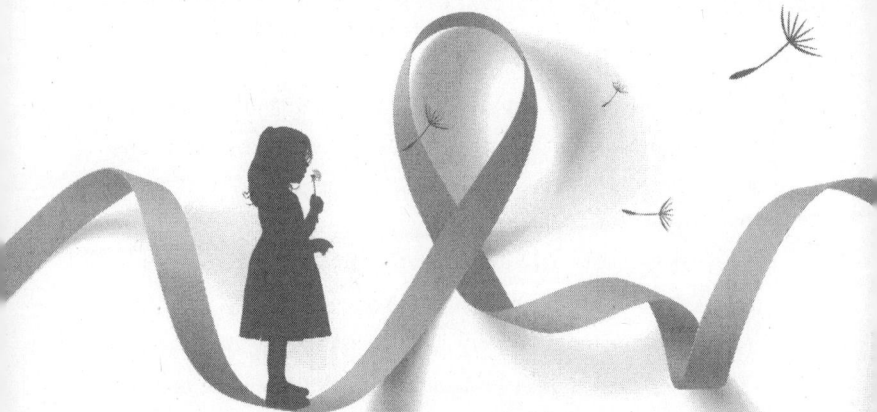

Lambor-buggy

Thursday 14th March 2019

My phone rings in my pocket; it is my younger sister, Sarah. She's in our #TeamLeah WhatsApp group, so she's well aware of what is going on and how Leah is, but she just wants to speak to me directly. Sarah is a qualified A&E nurse down in Birmingham and she's offered to travel up and do one or two of the overnight hospital stays with Leah to give Claire and I a break. Amy's overnight stay was a success, so I'm more than happy to accept Sarah's offer.

Sarah is desperate for us to be able to attend her wedding down in Lincoln in the middle of May. Leah and Phoebe are both due to be bridesmaids and Sarah is trying to understand whether they'll be able to make it.

I'd be lying if I said that this wasn't one of the things that had been on my mind over recent weeks. The wedding currently falls on a date between Leah's sixth and seventh scheduled chemotherapy rounds. It is impossible at this stage to know whether those rounds will commence on the dates planned. It is also impossible to know whether Leah's temperatures will mean that she is allowed out of hospital after round four is complete. It is also impossible to know whether Leah will be well enough or strong enough to attend a full-day event like that. It is also impossible to know whether we will be able to protect her sufficiently in an environment like that if her blood levels are dangerously low at that point. There are so many reasons why I cannot give my own sister a straight answer to whether or not her niece will be able to be one of her bridesmaids on the biggest day of her life. Sarah understands the situation and she puts no pressure on us, but, again, the reality of life for us kicks us in the ribcage one more time.

Friday 15th March 2019

The equipment ordered for Leah by the OT team arrived today. The armchair is chestnut brown and possibly the most aesthetically disappointing piece of furniture I've ever seen in my life. It does, however, have about fifty different levers and adjustment methods to allow it to be positioned in possibly three million different combinations, so I guess we can live with the chestnut brown (good old NHS).

Along with the armchair, we also take delivery of a large, foldable buggy. Leah is really struggling to walk far now and the standard wheelchair she has is too 'upright' for her to sit in for more than about ten minutes. Our hope is that the buggy will help her with that issue. She really doesn't like the thought of having to use a buggy as a six-year-old, but she is also hating the fact that she's been stuck in the house or in the hospital pretty much non-stop for the last six weeks. She might have to swallow her pride a little and see how the buggy goes.

The buggy has an aluminium frame and a detachable seat, which is bright blue. The seat reclines to any of a number of settings and is fairly easy to use. It looks really slick and quite expensive[21], like the Italian supercar version of a buggy. Given that it has a small Italian flag on the manufacturer's logo, that is probably not too far off the mark.

The early spring sun is shining outside, so we take the opportunity to try the new buggy out, and Leah and I take the dog for a walk around the estate where we live. Leah straps into the 'Lambor-buggy' like a racing driver, a baseball cap covering her threadbare scalp, and we leave the house together. It feels great to be out in the sunshine. I feel like I haven't felt that warmth for so long, both physically and metaphorically. Leah has clearly got over her issue with the buggy and she is smiling and chatting away to me as we walk up to the top of the hill overlooking the houses at the back of the estate.

Just to be able to get her out of the house and out for a walk in the sunshine makes such a positive difference to her morale as well as mine. For a few minutes, I sense perhaps the universe is trying to apologise for what has happened… and it feels beautiful.

---

21 I found the exact buggy via an internet search a few weeks later and it cost over £3,000 brand new!

Monday 18th March 2019

Since Leah returned home after the last round of chemo, she's been sleeping in the new bedroom that we've created for her. Either Claire or I are sleeping in the other bed in the room each night. This is far from ideal, but needs must, and it at least allows the other one of us to get some sleep. Whoever sleeps in Leah's room needs to set several alarms for a number of duties during the night. These include:

✓ Administering Leah's anti-sickness and pain medication at set intervals in accordance with the medicine schedule written on the whiteboard.
✓ Setting up her feed pump and ensuring it runs okay during the night to make sure she has adequate nutrition.
✓ Disconnecting her feed pump when the scheduled feed is complete.
✓ Taking her temperature with the digital thermometer in her ear each time any of the above tasks are carried out.

Claire was in with Leah last night and I slept in our bedroom. At about 2am, Claire walks into our room and wakes me up.

'Ste, Leah's temperature is high,' she says. This is not good news. We have been advised that a high temperature of 38°C or above, otherwise known as a spike in temperature, means that we need to bring her into hospital immediately for assessment, regardless of the day or time. I jump out of bed and follow Claire into Leah's room. Claire takes Leah's temperature again. Leah shuffles in her sleep as Claire places the thermometer probe into her ear. The thermometer beeps. The digital display flashes amber and the numbers on it read 38.2°C. We look at one another, both knowing what this means without having to say a word.

I agree to take Leah into the hospital, so I go back to our bedroom and get dressed. I throw a few basic toiletries and a change of clothes into a bag while Claire is doing the same for Leah. Within fifteen minutes, we've loaded the bags into the car, disconnected a sleepy Leah's feed pump, carried her downstairs and into the car, and I set off for the M62.

We arrive at Alder Hey about twenty minutes later and, after parking up, we make our way straight to the Accident & Emergency department. The hospital is eerily quiet at this time of night, although there are still a good few parents and children sat in the waiting room in A&E. I give Leah's details in at the reception desk and highlight that she is an oncology patient. One of the nurses on duty shepherds us into a small empty room behind reception, away from the main waiting room[22].

About ten minutes later, a nurse enters the room and asks whether she can do a set of observations on Leah. Leah is fast asleep on the trolley in the corner of the room and I'm dozing off in the chair next to her. It is now about

---

22 I found out later that this is a standard procedure for oncology
      patients with a raised temperature. They are isolated from others
      in order to minimise any risk of infection.

3am. The nurse takes Leah's blood pressure and oxygen saturation and then takes her temperature. 38.1°C. The nurse confirms the process from here on in. A small sample of blood will be taken from Leah's central line and sent to the lab to confirm her current blood count. If Leah's neutrophils are at a dangerously low level[23], she will be given a forty-eight-hour course of strong antibiotics to help her fight off any possible infection as quickly as possible. This, of course, means we'll be back in hospital for two days.

We get shown through to a cubicle in A&E and we stay there for an hour while we await the blood results. At around 4:30am, the blood results are confirmed. Her white cells are low. The porter comes shortly after to push Leah up to an empty room on Ward 3B and I follow behind.

I'm exhausted. Leah is already fast asleep. I message Claire to tell her what's going on. She messages me straight back, so she's not gone back to sleep properly either. It has been really nice being at home for the last four days or so. I'm now suspecting we may find that days at home could become the exception rather than the rule, though.

Wednesday 20th March 2019

The forty-eight-hour course of antibiotics came to an end early this morning and Leah's temperature is back under control, so we've been told she can return home at around lunchtime today. Unbelievably, her next round of chemotherapy is due to start tomorrow, so it doesn't really

---

23 Also known as neutropenic.

feel like a huge win getting back home today, but we'll all take it anyway.

The nursing team take a final blood sample from Leah's central line before we leave, so they can check that she is okay to commence tomorrow. By 1pm, we are safely back home and immediately working on re-packing the overnight bags.

Thursday 21st March 2019

Chemo round three was scheduled to start today. However, yesterday evening, we were told that the lab results from Leah's latest blood sample shows that Leah's blood count remains low. Essentially, her blood count has not recovered sufficiently from the impact of the previous round of chemo to make it safe for her to commence the next round. So, instead of making our way back to Alder Hey for the next three-day stint, the outreach team are coming to us to continue giving Leah the GCSF for a little longer.

The fact that her body already seems to be struggling to bounce back from the previous chemo is a slight cause for concern for me. It is probably not overly surprising given what she's been through this last week, though. At the end of the day, we really don't want her to have more treatment if she's not ready.

Friday 22nd March 2019

We get the lab results back from a blood sample taken this morning. Leah's bloods are much improved, so the plan is now for her to have the weekend off from any interventions and commence round three on Monday.

I have to say it's a relief on a personal level, but then again it means she's back in to have more poison pumped into her little body in three days' time and that is never going to be something to celebrate.

Saturday 23rd March 2019

It's Claire's birthday today. She categorically said that she didn't want any gifts or cards and she didn't want to go anywhere for the day. Personally, I kind of wanted us to try and get out somewhere with the girls and try to get a day's break from everything, but she is not at all in the headspace to do so. I understand that and it's her birthday, after all, so it's her call.

I bought a small gift for the girls to give to Claire and they come into our room first thing to sing happy birthday to her. This makes her smile, but it is as much as we celebrated. There is very little appetite for celebrating and having fun at the moment, while things are so serious for us and we have so much to think about.

Claire has disappeared out of view several times today and each time I've found her in our bedroom, sat on the bed, praying. Praying for Leah and for her mum. I know exactly what she really wants for her birthday. I also know that she'd probably trade in every gift she'll receive from now until the end of time to get that.

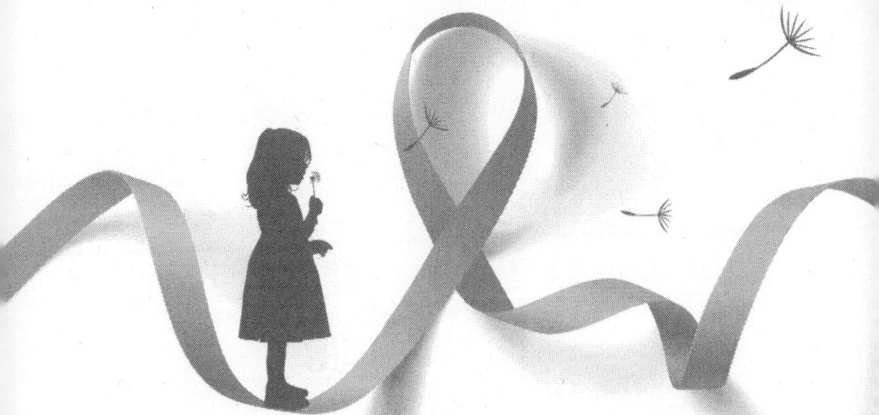

There's Always a Way

Marie is Claire's mum. My mother-in-law. I have to admit, as far as mother-in-laws go, I got pretty lucky. She's never been anything but wonderful to me and my family since the first day I gave Claire a lift home from work in my mum's old Ford Fiesta. She dotes on her kids and even more so on her grandkids, and the feelings are very much reciprocated. It was only very recently that I found out her name is Maria and not Marie. Everyone I know knows her as Marie. I've never quite got my head round that, if truth be told. I suppose it's just one of those strange, slightly older-generation things. For example, my own grandad was known all his life as Harry, but his real name was Joseph. It always makes me think of Trigger from *Only Fools and Horses*.

Marie was born in Uddingston, a town just outside Glasgow. I'd take a guess that you've never heard of the place, but if I told you that that's where the Tunnock's factory is (makers of foil-wrapped tea cakes and caramel wafers), I suspect it may be slightly more familiar. A proud Scot who has always stayed close to her roots, Marie has a kind heart and a fiery Celtic temperament to match, but only if you are silly enough to treat her wrong or support injustice and inequity. Marie is, without doubt, one of the best people I know at reading others and always stands up for the underdog. She is a Scottish sports fan at the end of the day, so it goes hand in hand.

As a child, Marie would regularly holiday on the Isle of Bute with her family. So, when she had the chance to buy her own little place on the island in later life, she jumped at it. I think it is her way of remaining connected to the places she loves the most, and we've all grown to love the island and the country in similar ways over time. Perhaps because Marie has promoted it so well. The Isle of Bute tourist board don't know what they've missed out on by not employing her.

One thing I always think about when I think of Marie is her incredible sense of positivity. She has never been one to dwell on the past or on the negative situations that happen throughout life. I've always found that personally quite inspiring and I've tried to instil that same attitude in my girls as they've grown up. Marie has a saying that she regularly uses to keep her, and others', spirits up: *There's always a way.*

Never have we all needed to remain positive as a family more than we do at the moment. Keeping Marie's saying in mind over recent months has become increasingly important. The irony is that the person who is best at keeping everyone around her upbeat is one of the ones facing the greatest challenges. I guess that's the art of being a great mum and grandmother, though. Carrying the burden for those you care for, often without them even knowing how heavy it is.

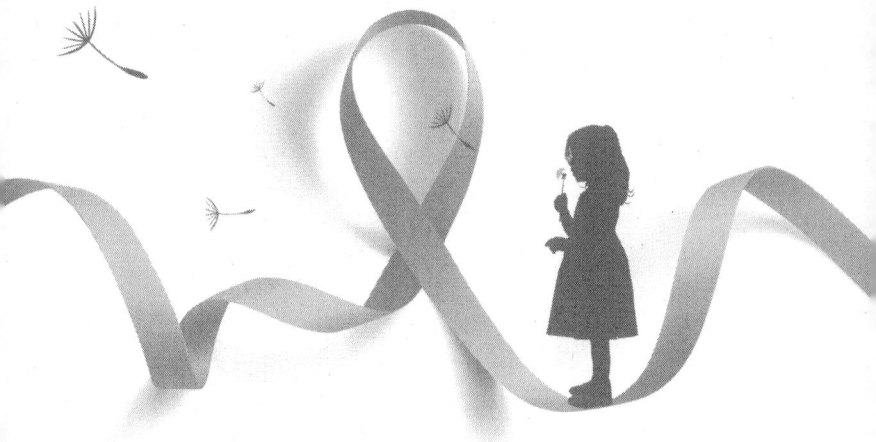

Princess Pilling

Monday 25th March 2019

We return to our second home at the hospital for the slightly delayed chemo round three to commence. After the impromptu early-morning trip to the hospital last week, Claire and I have agreed we need to be better prepared for regular hospital stays now. Therefore, we have packed a wheeled trolley with all the main items we need for an inpatient stay, along with a couple of bags for Leah and a bag for whoever is doing the overnight stay. Having this routine and the bags pre-packed will hopefully take a little of the stress away, as it means we are less likely to have forgotten to bring something that we really need. We are well on the way with our 'marathon' now, albeit still as very reluctant runners.

My mum and dad have collected Phoebe from school

and brought her to the hospital to see Leah. She has brought with her an A4 pink scrapbook and she hands it to Leah. The book has been created by Leah's classmates, who have been writing little stories in it and drawing her pictures to show they are thinking about her, to cheer her up.

Leah is thrilled to receive it and loves the quirky – some are very random – pictures that her friends have drawn for her. However, after she's read it, she looks a little dejected.

'What's up, Leah? Don't you like it?' Phoebe asks her. It transpires that this cute little gesture from her classmates has served to remind her just how much she misses them all and she asks whether she can go into school and see them. I'm not sure that this is a good idea, given Leah's current condition and the risks associated with her picking up an infection between treatment rounds, but I promise her I will look into it.

We've had another offer of help with the overnight hospital stays today from my cousin, Emma. She is currently training to be a paediatric nurse and has said she's happy to help out tonight as she has no university commitments tomorrow. Emma is Leah's godmother and Leah loves her to bits, so there are no complaints from that side. It gives Claire and I a night off, so it's a yes all round and Emma comes in to take over the reins just before we leave for the evening.

When we get home, I speak to Claire about the possibility of Leah going into school to visit her classmates. Claire shares my nervousness, but we agree it would be great for Leah's morale and agree to see if we can work with the school. I drop Leah's teacher, Mrs Harrison, an email to explain the situation and to see what she thinks. The school have been really supportive of our family since the devastation of Leah's initial diagnosis, but the truth is they don't really have any experience of how to handle a child with an illness like Leah's and they are generally much more nervous about things than we are. We shall see what they say.

Tuesday 26th March 2019

Day two of three for the third round of chemo and Leah is given a gift bag today courtesy of the Pippa Jones Little Treasure Trust. This is yet another small charity that I was previously unaware of. The bag contains a box containing a 'build your own princess crown' kit. Claire opens it up to try and encourage her to do something constructive. So far today, it is safe to say that she is not feeling the joy. She has a little go at sticking some plastic gems onto the pink, foam, tiara-like headband, but her heart clearly isn't in it.

A little later in the morning, Prof Pilling comes into the bay. He's conducting the ward round, reviewing all of the patients and checking on their progress since yesterday.

'Leah,' I say to her. 'Why don't you make your princess crown for Barry?' I'm half-joking, I suppose, but I'm also watching her reaction. She has a little glint of mischief in her eyes and she gives me a big smile. All of a sudden, the princess crown has a new purpose and she sits upright in her bed, frantically constructing the tiara before Barry reaches her bed.

About ten minutes later, he is just finishing up with his review of the young boy in the bed next to Leah when she declares her task complete. She has lined the outside of the tiara with blue and red 'gems' and there is a thick layer of silver glitter across the bottom. The words 'Princess Pilling' are proudly emblazoned across the front. She is so proud of what she has made and she is bouncing with excitement at the thought of handing over this most precious of gifts to him.

Barry approaches Leah's bed accompanied by the usual entourage of senior nurses and junior doctors.

'Hello, trouble,' he says to her. 'What have you been up to here?'

Leah shows him what she has made and one of his doctor colleagues says, 'It looks like she has made you your very own tiara, Barry. You're going to have to try it on now, aren't you?'.

There then follows a few seconds of awkward delay when none of us around the bed quite know whether how this is going to go.

Barry picks up the tiara, adjusts the size at the back and then proudly places it onto his head, prompting a light round of applause and some chuckles from the audience. I glance at Leah. She is laughing away with a big smile. It's a lovely moment and the first time I have sensed any kind of real connection between her and Barry.

Barry leaves the tiara on his head as he reviews Leah and he seems happy that all is in order and she's doing okay.

'I'm around the ward all day today, so I may see you later,' he says as he trundles off the bay and down the corridor to see the next patient. His bald head now has a light dusting of silver glitter. I chuckle to myself as I imagine him trying to be all serious and professional in the room next door with another family, while sparkling brightly.

Later in the afternoon, Claire and I are sat by Leah's bedside. Claire has dozed off on the small sofa, after having a busy night with Leah last night. Leah, too, has dozed off. I am sat flicking through my phone and I notice an email from Leah's schoolteacher, Mrs Harrison. She says it would be wonderful if Leah is able to come in and see her classmates, and that they will accommodate her visit on any day that suits her. I message her back to say that we'll try to bring her in on Friday, providing she gets out of hospital on time as planned and she is well enough in herself. She will love that.

I tell her when she wakes up an hour later and her smile says all I need to know. I really hope she can manage it. My excitement on her behalf is also tinged with anxiety. I desperately don't want to put her at risk in any way just so she can have a small amount of time back in the 'normal world'.

Wednesday 27th March 2019

Today is the final day of the latest round of chemotherapy. Leah has struggled physically these last three days, perhaps more than during any of the previous rounds of treatment. She has been really tired and has vomited a lot more this time. She has barely eaten a thing for three days either. The chemotherapy has completely taken away her appetite, yet she keeps trying to eat and nibbling small amounts every so often. We're already so proud of how she is coping with challenges that most adults would struggle with.

I think one of the main reasons she is managing to cope is because of the interaction she has with the staff on the ward. They treat her like a princess and always take time to chat with her and try to make her smile. It makes an enormous difference to her, and us, and keeps her spirits up.

Just after lunch today, an incredible lady called Georgina calls in to see Leah. Georgina is French and a professional cellist who plays in the Liverpool Philharmonic Orchestra. In her spare time, she is part of the 'music in hospitals' initiative and she spends an afternoon every week on the oncology ward playing music with the children. Georgina has Leah sat up in her bed, banging on a large drum, while she plays the theme tune from the *Harry Potter* films on her cello. I can't help but feel that these are precious moments and no matter what the future holds for Leah, I will never forget these moments – watching her playing the instruments and having fun. She is momentarily free from the darkness that has engulfed her life recently and that is simply priceless.

That evening, Marie and Peter come to visit. Marie is again in the wheelchair. She looks like she has lost even more weight since I saw her last and that could only have been a matter of days ago. If truth be told, she doesn't look well at all. But again, she is here and she is supporting us all. I just hope she starts to pick up soon and regains all the physical strength that seems to be steadily falling away from her.

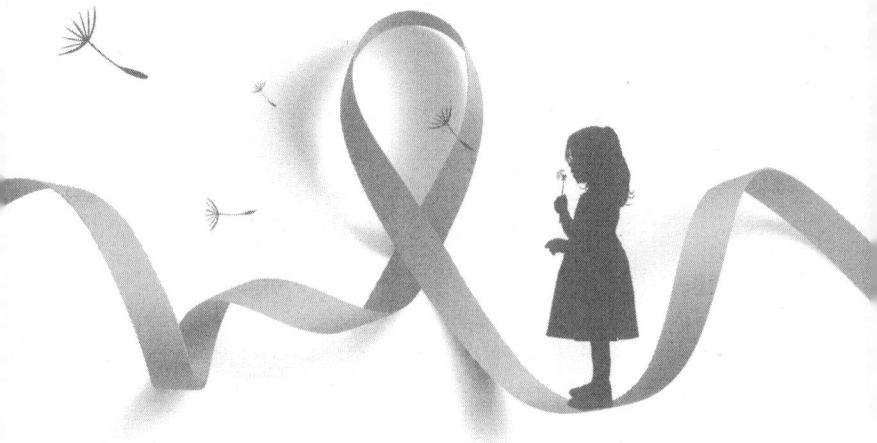

School Family

Thursday 28th March 2019

Leah is a little brighter when she wakes up and even manages a couple of spoonfuls of Rice Krispies. After her miniscule breakfast, she spends an hour in the ward classroom with Jo learning about the nations of the United Kingdom, their capital cities and famous landmarks.

The final drips of the chemotherapy drugs have been administered by early afternoon and, at around 4pm, we are told we can take her home. We never need telling twice; as soon as the bags are all packed, we are out of there and heading home. It feels good every time.

Friday 29th March 2019

Leah wakes up looking bright this morning. Possibly

because we're planning to take her into school to see her friends later on. She is super-excited about this. Since she started at school, she's always been on school dinners but consistently requested that we put her onto packed lunches... apart from on a Friday. On Friday, the school canteen makes fish and chips and it is Leah's absolute favourite meal of the week. Therefore, it is only fitting that the day she goes in to see her friends and classmates is 'Fishy Friday'.

Leah's teacher, Mrs Harrison, has helped plan the visit. We are to take her into the classroom at 11am and she can go and see all her classmates and chat to them all. Then she can choose five of her closest friends to have fish and chips with at lunchtime.

Leah is in good spirits and she seems reasonably well, so we take her into school at 11am as planned. She is a little reluctant to go in in her buggy. She doesn't really want her classmates to see her in it, but the reality is she is not able to sit for long periods of time in anything else, so it's the buggy or nothing!

Taking her in is incredibly emotional. Watching her smiling and laughing with her classmates is just beautiful – more beautiful than I imagined it would be. One by one, her classmates tell her what they've been doing over recent weeks and get her involved in the conversation, too. They tell her what they've been studying and they ask her what she's been doing in the hospital. Some of the other teachers and classroom assistants come in to see her and say hello. One or two of them are visibly struggling to hold back tears.

At midday, the rest of the class are led over to the canteen for their lunch. In the opposite direction comes one of the canteen staff wheeling a trolley with fish and chips on for Leah and her hand-picked gang of friends. The school have arranged for the children to eat in a small room adjacent to Leah's classroom. She doesn't eat much of the food, but it doesn't matter. For that hour in the classroom and the half an hour over lunchtime, she is not ill. She is not different. She is a pupil, a classmate, a friend. She has forgotten about her challenges, and Alder Hey feels like it is a million miles away.

Soon, it is time for us to go home. Leah is devastated. She desperately does not want to leave her friends behind and return to her other life. A life of hospital beds, bleeping drip stands, big red bags of poison and thermometers. However, we have to protect her and make sure she doesn't 'overdo' it. I know she understands that, but her tears in the back seat of the car on the way home weigh heavier on my heart than at any other time over the last few months.

Monday 1st April 2019

Today is a really exciting day! Alongside making arrangements for Leah to come into school to see her classmates, the school has also been asking about how they can show their support to Leah, Phoebe and the whole of our family. As a result, they have decided to arrange a 'Race for Life' fun run for the whole school to raise money for Cancer Research UK. Today is the day it is taking place.

All the children have been asked to dress in something pink and get sponsorship to run, jog or walk a mile. The school have arranged to have a path painted around the perimeter of the playground and a mile is essentially five laps of the path.

Leah was really pale when she woke up this morning. Her temperature was normal, but there was an element of us questioning whether it was the right thing to do to take her into school to join in or not. There are occasions when the risk of her picking up an infection is sometimes outweighed by the negative impact on her morale if we stop her from doing something that she desperately wants to do. It regularly feels like a near impossible balancing act. The whole event today will be outside on the school playground, so the risks of her picking something up are reduced. Claire and I both agree we should take her along.

We arrive a little later than planned at the school. My mum and dad are already there, along with my older sister, Deb, and Claire's sister, Amy. All the kids look amazing, with flashes of pink clothing everywhere. A few of them have even made T-shirts with #TeamLeah emblazoned on the front. It's really quite emotional to be standing here and feeling such overwhelming support for the girls.

Leah doesn't have the strength to run, jog or walk a mile at the moment, so we agree that she can take part as long as she lets Claire or I push her round the course in her buggy. Reluctantly, she agrees. However, as soon as we set off on the first lap, all the kids from her class surround her and run alongside us. Leah is shouting and laughing with them all and lapping up the attention.

In true Leah style, after completing four of the five laps, she insists on getting out of the buggy and completing the last lap alongside her friends and definitely without Claire or I. Cautiously, we agree, and then watch as she jogs off, holding hands in a chain with about six others. I watch her jogging and skipping her way round the path, my heart bursting with pride. The fighting spirit she has shown over the last couple of months, the same spirit she will need for the months ahead, is just oozing out of her. Her determination to overcome the obstacles and succeed is quite simply incredible for someone her age. It fills me with hope that maybe, just maybe, she has what it takes to overcome this. I know in my heart that whatever happens over the next few months and whatever the future holds for her, she will one hundred per cent not fail because of a lack of spirit or fight on her part.

The only negative aspect of a fabulous afternoon is that Marie and Peter didn't come along. Marie messaged Claire in the morning to say she wasn't feeling up to it, but she wished us all the best of luck. Hell and high water would not have kept Marie away from this event today and the opportunity to support her daughter and granddaughters. It is a real worry.

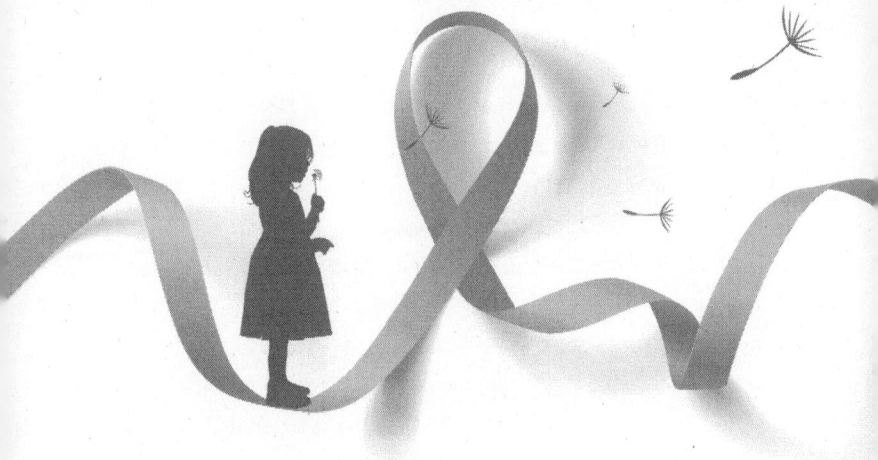

Spaceships and Magpies

Wednesday 3rd April 2019

Today is yet another big day for us. They just keep on coming, don't they? It is the day of Leah's next MRI scan. The first she has had since she commenced the chemotherapy. After the scan, we just have to sit and wait for the results… and keep absolutely everything crossed that they are positive. The results will inform us whether the chemo treatment is doing its job and shrinking this thing in her body. I can't even think about the scenario where this is not happening.

In the waiting room of the radiology department at the hospital, one of the staff helps apply numbing cream to the backs of Leah's hands and the areas on the bend of her arms opposite her elbows. The numbing cream should help when they come to inject the contrast dye into her body for the final few images. That is the bit Leah is most frightened of. However, when the time comes for that to happen, she actually deals with it fairly well and allows them to do the injection.

Claire and I sit at the foot of the scanner. Claire prays continuously for the duration of the scan again and, I must admit, even I close my eyes and ask the Big Guy Upstairs for some help this time. He probably won't listen to me as I haven't really spoken to him since I was a kid at Sunday School, but I suppose I have to start rebuilding this relationship at some point, so why not now?

Thursday 4th April 2019

It is a beautiful, fresh early spring morning. A little on the chilly side, but the sunlight is bursting through the windows when I wake up. It makes me feel positive and uplifted.

At around 11:30am, my mobile phone rings. 'No Caller ID' is displayed across the screen. That usually means it is someone from Alder Hey.

'Hello?' I answer.

'Hello, it's Barry Pilling here,' the gruff voice on the other end responds.

I can't really explain why, but just hearing Prof. Pilling's voice makes me stop dead in my tracks and makes me anxious. In my heart, I know he is just doing his job, but, at the same time, this man has said things to me that have broken me into pieces and I have that association with his voice now. I take a deep breath in.

'Hi, Barry,' I reply. *It's about time you gave us some positive news now, Barry – so come on, let's hear it.*

Barry informs me that the oncology team have fast-tracked the results from Leah's scan yesterday. My heart starts racing and the knot in my stomach suddenly feels tighter than usual. Despite three rounds of intensive and fairly destructive chemotherapy, the tumour on Leah's spine does not appear to have gotten any smaller in size. I close my eyes and bow my head. My phone almost slips from my hand as my grip goes weak. Claire is stood right alongside me, desperately trying to gauge my reaction. Judging by the look of anguish on her face, she's already worked out what I've just been told.

Our main hope of getting a successful outcome for our little girl rests on the ability of the chemotherapy to shrink the tumour and therefore make the challenge of surgically removing it slightly less complicated or risky. That hope has faded drastically in the last thirty seconds.

Prof Pilling goes on to tell me that he is disappointed with the results and has already discussed whether to continue the chemo treatment beyond the initial three rounds, given the seemingly poor response. He tells me that he has discussed this with Professor Bernadette Bannan from Central Manchester Children's Hospital. In Barry's opinion, she is the best in the country when it comes to paediatric sarcomas.

Prof. Bannan has suggested to Barry that there may be benefits to continuing with the treatment on the hope that the effects of the chemo may be cumulative. Therefore, Barry is comfortable with a decision to continue with the treatment for three further rounds and then see whether the next MRI scan shows a more positive impact. The next scan has been provisionally booked for the end of May. Barry then confirms that Leah's next round of chemo will start on Tuesday next week, before he wishes us a pleasant weekend and ends the call. There is silence in the room.

Claire and I are trying to process the information we've just been given. We're obviously relieved to hear that they are planning to continue treatment, but there is no doubt that, overall, the news of the scan result is not what we wanted to hear. Still, while Leah has a treatment plan, we have continued hope and it is that which allows us to keep going and giving our best to Leah, to Phoebe and to each other. We desperately need to cling onto any hope we can.

Saturday 6th April 2019

In all the madness that has surrounded our lives over recent months, we've almost lost sight of the fact that Leah and Phoebe are scheduled to be bridesmaids at my sister's wedding in May. I have worked out that the wedding falls just after the planned completion of chemo round six – that is, providing there are no material delays to any of the next rounds. At this point in time, I still have absolutely no idea whether Leah will be well enough to travel down and take part, but we try to stay positive and optimistic that she will manage it. Sarah's wedding is one of the few points of light that we have at the moment. We know we need to do everything in our power to make sure the girls get there and have an amazing day.

Leah has been understandably worried about how she will look at the wedding and on the wedding photos in particular. Generally, the loss of her hair hasn't bothered her too much, as she knows it will grow back when her treatment has finished, but she hates the thought that she might look bald and ill in front of a lot of strangers. Therefore, Claire has been in touch with the Little Princess Trust[24] over the last few weeks to see whether they might be able to provide Leah with a wig for the wedding. Last week, the charity got back in touch to confirm that they could help and we have an appointment later today at a wig shop in Liverpool to get her measured and fitted.

When we arrive, the lady working in the wig shop makes a huge fuss of Leah. She makes her feel really special. Leah tries on a few different wigs to get as close to her natural hair colour as possible. None of the wigs are the perfect size to fit her scalp and they are all long in length, so they don't really suit her perfectly. Leah is having fun swishing the hair round and posing in the mirror. Eventually, we agree the right size and the best match we can get on the colour.

It is another day of fighting back emotion for me. This little girl is six years old. She shouldn't have to need a wig just so that she feels comfortable at her aunt's wedding. She shouldn't have to go through these experiences at all. But she does, and she does them all with a smile on

---

24 The Little Princess Trust is an incredible charity who accept donations from wonderful people all over the country who choose to grow out, then chop off and donate their hair to be turned into real-hair wigs for children undergoing treatment like Leah.

her face and a determination that never fails to make me proud.

The wig for the wedding is now ordered. We agree with the shop owner that it will be shortened to shoulder-length and then delivered to our house the week before the wedding in early May. All of the costs are covered by the Little Princess Trust, so we don't have to worry about how to pay for it[25]. Claire will then arrange for the local hairdressers to style the hair as Leah would like for the wedding. We just need to keep everything crossed that we can get her there now.

Tuesday 9th April 2019

Leah's blood count, as taken by the outreach team yesterday, is back within the safe levels. Therefore, we are back at Alder Hey, complete with a car full of bags, as chemotherapy round four commences. This round of treatment is the IE drugs and this stay is another six-day stint. Leah is again attached by tubes to the drip stand that will follow her everywhere she goes for the next six days, beeping and flashing relentlessly like some kind of annoying Dalek.

At lunchtime, I decide to take a wander down to the hospital canteen to get something decent to eat. Something other than a microwave meal for one. While walking to the canteen, I notice a familiar programme playing on one of the TVs in the waiting areas. It is a cartoon called *Ben &*

---

25 It is estimated to cost, on average, £600 to supply a single child with a wig.

Holly's Little Kingdom. This is a cartoon that both Phoebe and Leah loved watching when they were younger.

One of the less common characters in the programme is a large fish that causes chaos to some of the other characters by eating their boats. The fish is called Big Bad Barry. While standing in the food queue in the canteen, my thoughts turn to Prof. Pilling. Our very own Big Bad Barry. So far he's chewed up and spat out every single boatload of positivity that we've managed to scrape together. I wonder whether the cartoon character is actually based on him – obviously minus the suit and trainers.

Wednesday 10th April 2019

I stayed in the hospital with Leah last night and it was yet another tough night. This time, though, my concerns do not centre around Leah, but the little boy in the bed next to her.

The night from Leah's perspective was fairly uneventful. I managed to get a handful of crisps down her and a reasonable drink of full fat milk before we read a few chapters of *Fantastic Mr Fox* and she fell asleep at around 10pm. I was tired myself and settled down to sleep soon after. At that point, the bed next to Leah was empty.

At around 1:30am, I am woken by the sounds of people in the adjacent bed space. By the look of things, someone else has had to bring their child into the hospital unexpectedly in the early hours. However, it is apparent that this little boy has not simply been brought in with a high temperature as a precaution. The poor kid sounds awful and is audibly struggling to breathe.

There is a lot of activity around the bed space throughout the night, with doctors and nurses popping in and out. I am trying hard to switch off from the noise and get some sleep, but I can't help but be concerned for the boy. It sounds like his oxygen levels are worryingly low and he is being given oxygen directly through a mask. His breathing difficulties continue for a few hours. It transports me right back to the night in late February when Leah was in real pain with her kidneys. This is how the other families on the ward that night must have felt. I dearly want to reach out and help that little boy and his family, but I know there is nothing I can do. Eventually, fatigue gets the better of me and I fall asleep.

When I wake in the morning, the curtain is pulled round the little boy's bed. I have no idea who this family are and who this boy is, but I was genuinely really frightened for them all last night and I was fearful for what I would wake up to this morning. It sounds like the medical and nursing teams must have managed to stabilise him at some point. I can hear light snoring, which suggests whoever is behind the curtain is asleep. This is a relief.

Later in the day, Claire comes in to see Leah and to take over from me for the rest of the afternoon and the evening. I am just starting to pack my things together when a short, auburn-haired lady in glasses approaches the bed.

'Hello, my name is Tracy. Would you like a story?' she asks Leah.

Leah has been fairly quiet all morning. I presume this is because her sleep was disturbed during the night through a combination of noise from the next bed and the usual regular toilet treks. However, she agrees to the offer of a story, so Tracy makes herself comfortable next to the bed and, with her eyes fixed on Leah, she begins.

The story is a Russian folk tale of a witch called Baba Yaga who threatens to eat children. Despite the fairly dark content, Tracy has her audience completely transfixed and engaged with the tale. Even Leah was listening intently! I watch her as she interacts with Tracy, who describes the story so well without reading from a book, and Leah hangs on her every word.

The story goes on for about ten minutes and, at the end, Leah is left smiling and energised. These small moments that break up the mundanity of the long hospital stays are priceless in terms of helping to keep the kids' spirits up. Six days feels like such a long time for me, so six days of feeling sick and not being able to go much further than the end of your bed must feel like an eternity for Leah. Having the ability to whisk a child away into a fairy-tale world for just ten minutes and help them forget their troubles is an underrated superpower in my eyes. For information, no children were eaten during the performance.

Thursday 11th April 2019

Seconds out, round four, day three – ding, ding. Leah seems to be struggling more with this round of chemo than any of the previous ones in terms of her tolerance for the drugs. She's vomiting a lot and Claire and I have agreed to back away from trying to push her to eat food. There doesn't seem to be much to gain at the moment to balance out the unnecessary strain it puts on our relationship with her. Even the milk via her feed pump is coming back up at regular intervals.

Later in the morning, Ian – another of the advanced nurse practitioners on the ward – comes over to review Leah and check how she's getting on. He agrees that we perhaps shouldn't push her to eat while she's struggling to hold anything down.

'It won't do her any harm for a day or so,' he advises. My concern is that 'a day or so' can easily turn into weeks and I'm desperate to try and help her keep her strength up. To do that, she needs to be eating something.

After Ian completes his review, he pulls a small yellow carboard box out of his pocket and hands it to Leah. The box contains a small amount of Lego[26]. He then wanders over to the young boy in the bed next to her and hands him a box, too. It turns out the boy's name is Jacob and he is the child who was struggling to breathe a couple of nights ago. Thankfully, he seems to be doing much better now. Ian sets Leah and Jacob a challenge to build the best model they can in ten minutes, after which time he will come back and judge whose model is best. Leah, being an incredibly determined and very competitive young lady, has got her game face on and she is already flinging various bits of Lego around frantically to create her masterpiece. I glance across to Jacob's bed and he appears to be taking this challenge equally as seriously as Leah.

---

26 The boxes of Lego are donated to the ward by a charity called Fairy Bricks.

For ten minutes, Leah and Jacob have completely forgotten that they are in hospital. Leah is hooked up to the large red bags of poison and Jacob, who was fighting to breathe a day or so ago, seem to be completely oblivious to their own situations. I glance across to Jacob's dad and smile. He smiles back and gives a small nod of appreciation. I can tell he is grateful for this moment, too. Either that or he's thinking 'My son is about to kick your daughter's arse in this competition'.

About twenty minutes later, Ian returns to the bay for the grand judging. Leah has built a small multicoloured house. Jacob has built a spaceship. If I'm brutally honest, Jacob's spaceship is a clear winner (I think his dad knows that, too). This kid is obviously no stranger to a box of Lego. Ian, however, has obviously judged these types of competitions many times and declares it a draw. Both of them are given a chocolate Freddo as a prize and both seem to be accepting of that outcome, although I suspect Jacob is feeling a little hard done by.

Just after lunchtime, Prof Pilling swings by and invites Claire and I into one of the consultation rooms at the top of the ward. We follow him in and sit down opposite him at the desk. My heart is thumping again. It does every time I speak to him. He begins by telling us that he is intending to take her case to a national sarcoma MDT at the end of the month. He wishes to gauge the views of oncology and surgical teams from a network of other paediatric oncology departments across the country. I interpret this as a positive, as it could potentially open up further treatment opportunities for Leah from other parts of the country if required.

He then informs us that he has been discussing Leah's case with surgical colleagues at the hospital to explore the possibility of surgery. He tells us that, at this point in time, the feedback from the surgeons is that they are extremely sceptical about attempting surgery. They believe it may be far too risky and probably has a very limited chance of success.

Ouch. Hearing that hurts… it really hurts. With those words alone, the faint light at the end of this seemingly huge tunnel just got significantly dimmer.

Big Bad Barry strikes again, eh?

Friday 12th April 2019

I find it quite strange and a little unnerving that we still seem to be waiting to hear the results of the scan Marie had a few weeks ago. I'm fairly sure she had an appointment with her consultant at the Clatterbridge Cancer Centre earlier this week, but Claire hasn't mentioned anything.

Amy has agreed to cover tonight in the hospital for us, which, again, is hugely appreciated. She arrives at the hospital just after 7pm and I start packing my bag and gathering up Leah's dirty washing to take home.

'Sorry I'm late,' she says to me. 'I've just been round Mum and Dad's.'

'Oh, how is your mum?' I ask.

'She's okay,' Amy replies.

She seems quite quiet and a little distracted, so I ask her if she's sure she's okay to do the night.

'Yes, of course, you go home. We'll be fine,' she says as she smiles gently at Leah.

Leah, despite vomiting a lot over the last few days, seems settled. She also seems pleased by the fact that Auntie Amy is staying with her tonight. I pick up the bags, give Leah a kiss and wish them both a good night.

As I drive home along the motorway, I reflect on the metaphorical journey we're on and where we currently are. The whole thing is just relentless. It is both emotionally and physically draining. A night away from the hospital to spend together with Claire and Phoebe is really welcome. I feel relieved, but also strangely content. Content that while this whole thing is incredibly challenging, I do feel that we're dealing with it as best we can. With the help of so many people, it feels like we are just about coping. I'm proud of that and I'm proud of the people around us who are all playing their part – #TeamLeah. I allow myself to smile, but it quickly turns into a yawn.

Monday 15th April 2019

At long last, the final day of this mammoth six-day stint has arrived. This has been, without doubt, the toughest one yet for Leah. She is exhausted and she's been really unwell for the majority of the time in hospital. We are desperate to get her home and, all being well, she will be discharged later this afternoon and Claire will bring her back.

It's the Easter holidays from school, so Phoebe is off and I agree to take her swimming. It is the first time we've been swimming since the week before Leah's diagnosis and the first time I've been with just one of the girls since they were babies. In hindsight, I'm not too sure it was a good decision to come. It is really hard being here without Leah. It just feels wrong. Imbalanced in some way.

My brain starts to wander and I think about the worst scenarios again. The fact is, it is looking more and more likely that I may never get to bring both my girls swimming again. This imbalance could become permanent. Thankfully, I don't think Phoebe noticed how ridiculously emotional I was getting or how much I was struggling. I'm glad I don't have to explain myself to her and it turns out that it is quite easy to hide wet eyes in a swimming pool.

On the way home, I notice something strange out of the window. All of a sudden, there seems to be a lot of large birds appearing at the side of the road and in the trees around me. Specifically magpies. Perhaps they've always been there and I just haven't noticed them before? They suddenly seem to be on every hedgerow and tree with low branches on both sides of the road.

The thing is, they are all single magpies. 'One for sorrow' and all that. I've never really considered myself to be superstitious – in fact, I've always scoffed at things like that in the past. But, suddenly, I keep seeing single magpies bloody everywhere! Is this the universe trying to rub my nose in it? I start looking desperately for two magpies together. Come on! I need 'two for joy'. No such luck. The closest I got was seeing one at the end of the road to our house and another soon after sat on the aerial of the house next door to ours. Surely they are close enough to count as two together?

I did say I was desperate.

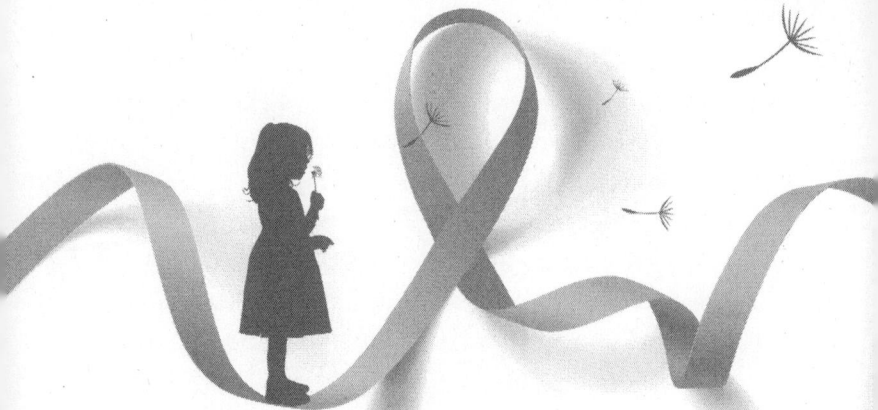

Warriors

Tuesday 16th April 2019

Claire left the house quite early this morning to go and see her mum and Dad. I haven't heard from her since she left. Leah has slept for most of the last twenty-four hours on and off, which shows how much the last six days have taken out of her. It's easy for me to have a moan about how emotionally and physically exhausting this whole thing is for me, but I always come back to thinking about Leah and how difficult it must be for her. She doesn't get the choice to have a night off or even to sleep in her own bed without being disturbed for even a single night. She gets up every day and fights on. I'm unbelievably proud of her.

The term 'warrior' is often used to describe people going through cancer treatment. The treatment regime is also frequently referred to as a 'battle'. Not everyone likes these terms or relates to them, but I think I do. I see the 'battle' every day with my own eyes. People not only fighting the physical impact of the treatments, but, perhaps more powerfully, facing up to the emotional struggle. Day after day. Week after week. Without any real breaks.

Leah is undoubtedly a warrior in my eyes, and so is Marie. The pair of them deal with everything this disease is throwing at them and somehow find the spirit and tenacity to keep on going. To keep taking the drugs that make them sick while trying to make them better. To keep eating the food that they don't have any appetite for and makes them feel sick, because they know if they don't, it will make them worse. These cancer warriors are special people. They have the hearts of lions and I am humbled to have two of them in my life right now. They constantly make me realise that I have nothing to moan about.

Later in the afternoon, Claire returns home. She walks through the door and comes into the living room where I'm sat. I can tell the second she enters the room that she is upset. She has concern written all over her face.

'What's the matter, baby?' I ask her. 'What's wrong?'

'It's my mum. She's had her scan results back and it's spread. It's spread everywhere! Oh God, Ste, she looks so poorly.'

I close my eyes and bow my head. I feel sick. I hold Claire close while she sobs into my shoulder. I don't know what to say. How the hell do we deal with this? How do I support Claire? How does Claire support her mum, her dad and her sister with everything else we have going on right now? How is this fair? How on earth did we get here?

Claire tells me she doesn't know what the treatment plan for her mum is from here. She doesn't know what drugs they will try next for her. I know in my heart that this is fast becoming a desperate situation, but I hope there are more options for Marie to try and I hope even more that she has the strength to try more options. A weary warrior is going to have to trudge into yet another battle.

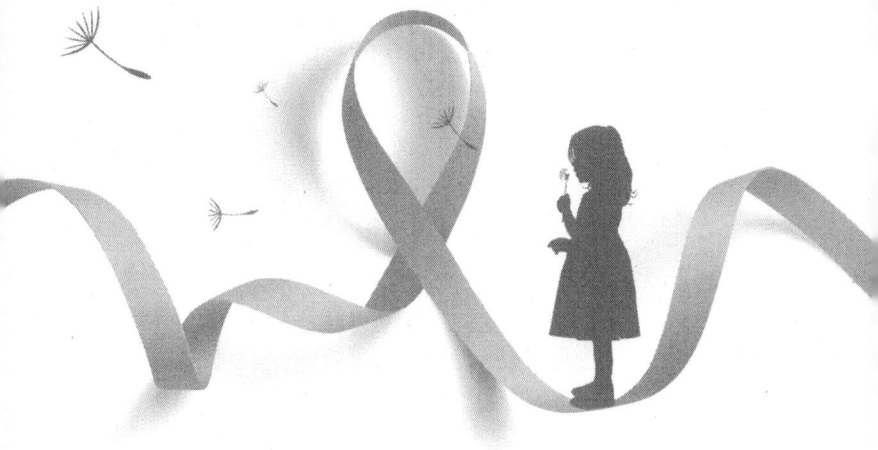

Charities, Large and Small

There is a famous motivational quote that people often reel off when they are dealing with difficult times: *When it rains, look for rainbows. When it's dark, look for stars.*

It's a classic 'easier said than done' statement and many people in the eye of a particular personal storm will find it hard to comprehend. There are certainly moments during these last few months when I've really, really struggled to find any rainbows or even a single star. However, on reflection, they are definitely there and they always have been. Many of those rainbows and shining stars come in the form of support from various charities. Organisations, large and small, whose sole purpose is to provide moments of light to kids like Leah and families like ours in their darkest days.

Within a week of Leah's first hospital stay at Alder Hey, one of the senior nurses on the ward handed us a large royal-blue canvas holdall. Apparently, all new families on the ward are given one of these bags. The bag contained a toilet bag stuffed with toothpaste, soap, a flannel and some shower gel. It also contained a small light-blue woollen beanie hat (to cover a little bald head); a home-made, knitted elephant teddy; a digital thermometer for regular temperature checking; a neck pillow (presumably for when you have to sleep in a chair); a beautiful rainbow-coloured fleece blanket; and a large bag of Jelly Babies.

These bags are created and donated by a small charity called Milly's Smiles based in Lancashire. Milly's Smiles was set up by a local family who lost their daughter, Milly, to cancer a few years previous. Receiving the bag reminded me that we were not alone in this strange world we found ourselves in. Many other families have trodden this difficult path before us and, sadly, many more will follow. That feeling of not being alone gave me some comfort and the fact that someone had gone out of their way to give us this bag (as well as donate money to create it in the first place) was incredibly humbling. The contents were exactly what we needed to help us on the journey ahead and could only have been created by someone who had walked this walk in the past. That bag was most definitely a star twinkling in the darkness.

In an earlier chapter, I mentioned Nugget from CLIC Sargent – a charity that funds staff to provide day-to-day support to young people diagnosed with cancer and their families. They help ensure families are able to access financial support and assist them with completing some of the paperwork required. CLIC Sargent – or Young Lives vs Cancer, as they are now known – are most definitely a rainbow in a stormy grey sky.

Tracy, the auburn-haired storyteller who came to see Leah on the ward, was funded by another local charity called Henry Dancer Days. This charity pay for wonderful and energetic people like Tracy to come and tell stories and sing songs to children in hospital with serious conditions. The result of this was to magically whisk Leah away to a different place for a few minutes with a story. For that few minutes, we were all able to forget our difficulties and negativity that can easily consume you.

I'll also never forget the day that a parcel arrived at home for Leah. Inside was a bright red shoebox with Converse written on the side. She lifted the lid and inside was a beautiful pair of hand-painted canvas ankle boots – the trainers she had designed back in March with Nugget had finally arrived. They had her name painted on the backs, a large rainbow painted on the side of one and a pug on the side of the other, just as Leah had requested. They looked fantastic and she was beaming as she climbed out of bed and put them on for the first time with her pyjamas. Her very own, personally designed Supershoes, hand-painted by a super talented artist and paid for by a super unique little charity.

When I stop and think about it now, our dark sky was actually littered with shining stars. Moments of love and positivity and kindness. Tiny moments that made an incredible difference and were, on occasion, the thing that kept us going. Many of the charities we encountered will be unknown to the vast majority of people, but if you find yourself with a spare few minutes after reading this book, please take a second to find out more about these incredible charities doing such important work. I wish that they did not need to exist, but they do, and if you ever find yourself having to follow this difficult journey, these organisations will walk alongside you:

Alder Hey Children's Charity
The Clatterbridge Cancer Charity
Beads of Courage UK
CLIC Sargent (now known as Young Lives vs Cancer)
Fairy Bricks
Ronald McDonald House
Pyjama Fairies
The Pippa Jones Little Treasure Trust
Supershoes
Little Princess Trust
Henry Dancer Days
Family Fund
Kids Cancer Charity
Milly's Smiles
Macmillan Cancer Support
Merlin's Magic Wand
Liverpool CHICS
End of Treatment Bells
When You Wish Upon A Star
Barrie Wells Trust
Owen McVeigh Foundation

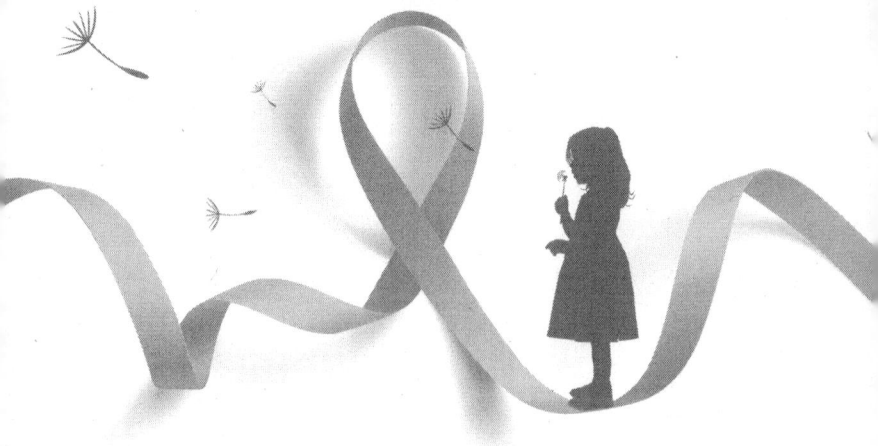

In Her Best Interests

Saturday 20th April 2019

Marie's health seems to be deteriorating quite rapidly. We took the girls round to see her on Thursday evening and she was asleep for the vast majority of our visit. Claire is trying to keep a brave face on and continuing to think positively, but I'm not sure whether the true magnitude of the situation has dawned on her yet. She's gone round to her mum and dad's again today and she's been there most of the day. I've stayed at home and made sure Leah has had all her meds on time. I've also tried my best to get bits of food down her periodically throughout the day, with varying degrees of success.

The clock ticks past 9:30pm and Claire still isn't home, so I drop her a text message to let her know that I'm putting the girls to bed and that I'm thinking of her. She doesn't reply. By the time the girls are settled in bed, it has gone 10:45pm. I've started Leah's feed pump for the night and taken her temperature. She's already asleep so I take the opportunity to jump in the shower before bed. I can't stop thinking about Claire, about Marie, about Peter and then about Leah. Everything feels like a blur. Like a bad dream, but, sadly, I know it's real.

At about 11:15pm, I hear Claire's car pull onto the drive and then her key turn in the front door. She comes straight up the stairs and into our bedroom, where I'm sat on the bed, watching TV.

'She's dying, Ste. My mum is dying!' she whimpers.

Her eyes are red and puffy and her mascara has been smeared across her left cheek. All I can see is the look of defeat on her face, the look of dejection and despair.

I jump up from the bed and throw my arms around her. 'I'm so sorry, honey.'

What else can I possibly say? My wife is completely heartbroken and I cannot do anything to make it better. I cannot fix it for her. I break down on her shoulder, too, and the pair of us just stand there in tears for what feels like forever.

Eventually, we sit on the bed and talk together for an hour or so. Claire talks to me about her mum and the fact that it is now clear that her life is coming to an end. But, perhaps more importantly, the fact that after more than two years of battling away, Marie herself is now fully accepting of her fate and has seemingly made peace with it.

Such is the level of cruelty in our current situation that, at around 1am, I need to say goodnight to Claire and go into Leah's room to undertake the usual 'night duties'. I have little choice but to kiss her on the forehead and leave her to deal with this alone. Just as I'm about to leave the room, she touches my arm, stares directly into my eyes and tells me one final thing.

'My mum said to me tonight...' She pauses. 'My mum said to me tonight that she knows she can't be saved...' I see her eyes welling up once more. 'But she is praying that losing her fight will mean that Leah might be saved. She is happy to give her own life for that of her granddaughter.'

I have no words to respond to this. Wow. Just... wow. I kiss her once more and go into Leah's room. I lie awake for at least two hours thinking about what Claire said. I have goosebumps at the thought of it. It feels huge. The biggest offer of help that anyone could ever give us. Is that really a choice she is able to make, though?

Thursday 25th April 2019

Today marks the start of Leah's next round of chemotherapy – round five. Thankfully, given everything that is happening in our family right now, it is only a three-day stay in hospital. I dearly wish this could be delayed or postponed so we could all focus on Marie, but we all know how important it is that we maintain Leah's treatment regime.

I've offered to cover all three nights while Marie is so unwell, so Claire can spend time with her family, but she is insisting that she needs to spend time with Leah, too. Therefore, we agree I will cover tonight and Saturday, and Claire will cover tomorrow. We've been told that Marie probably only has a matter of weeks to live. Peter, Claire and Amy are adamant that they will ensure she has someone at her bedside 24/7. The next few days and weeks are about to get tougher than I can even begin to imagine. I don't have the first idea how to manage this and I only hope we can all find the strength from somewhere to ride out this latest enormous storm.

Friday 26th April 2019

Big Bad Barry is taking Leah's case to the national sarcoma MDT for discussion at some point today. It has taken somewhat of a back seat in the melee that has surrounded us at home with Marie's situation, but it's impossible to forget it completely. The reality is that a positive discussion and outcome from this meeting could be Leah's only real chance of getting through this.

I feel a huge amount of anxiety around the MDT discussion. It feels like we have zero control over a decision that is possibly the most important of our entire lives. I know we won't hear any feedback today, but I dearly wish I could be a fly on the wall in the conversation. Even better, I wish we were allowed to be part of the conversation, but that apparently is not how this thing works… crazily, it doesn't seem to matter what Mum and Dad's views and wishes are.

Claire is at her mum and dad's again today. Later on, she will have to leave her mum's bedside after nursing her through one of her final days of life due to cancer. Then she will drive to the hospital and sit by her six-year-old daughter's bedside and nurse her through chemotherapy treatment for the same disease. This is painfully difficult for all of us, but I can only imagine how tough this must be for Claire. This is a situation that nobody should ever, ever have to deal with in their life. It feels so cruel and surreal.

I'm starting to see really clearly where Leah gets her strength and determination from though. I've never been prouder of Claire. I don't quite know how she is able to function right now. She's like Superwoman. Fuelled by love for two of the most important people in her life and her desire to support them as best she can. I don't think she realises that her strength is powering me through at the moment, too. I just don't want to let her down.

Sunday 28th April 2019

Leah's fifth round of chemo comes to an end. Her temperature has been steady over the last three days, so I'm confident she'll be okay to come home later today. I spoke to Claire on the phone earlier. Marie is now completely bed-bound and looking extremely weak. She is sleeping a lot. The whole situation is really distressing for Claire and her family, as it is just so unlike the Marie that we all know. It breaks my heart to think of a woman who has been so strong throughout her life being barely able to get out of bed, unable to eat a reasonable portion of food and unable to hold a conversation for more than about ten minutes. This disease is evil. It is seemingly stealing the lives and the dignity of people I love and yet none of us can do a thing about it. How can that be fair? These are good people! How can this be right?

As I'd hoped, Leah is allowed to go home after her treatment finishes, so, just after 3pm, we are handed the usual bag of medicines and a discharge letter, and we gather our bags and make our way to the car park.

We arrive home around thirty minutes later and what is sat on the roof of our porch to greet us as we travel up the drive? Yes, a bloody magpie. *One* magpie. I swear to God if I only had a shotgun…

Monday 29th April 2019

We've brought the girls round to see Claire's mum and dad today. It is the first time I've seen Marie for a good few weeks and, I'll be honest, I was more than a little nervous coming round. I know she's really unwell at the moment, but I didn't know what to expect and really don't want to get upset in front of her, especially seeing as she has been so strong in front of the rest of us over these last few years.

We go into the house and up to her bedroom. Marie is lying in bed. Peter is sat on the bed next to her. I notice he is holding her hand and I feel the lump in my throat already.

'Hi, Gran,' shouts Phoebe and goes over to give her a kiss on the head.

Marie gives her a faint smile and says, 'Hi, Phoebe,' in a very hushed tone. It seems like she even struggled to get those words out.

'Hi, Leah. Hi, Ste,' she follows.

She looks pale and tired. She is clearly very unwell, but she actually looks better than the image I had conjured up in my head before I came. Leah is really quiet. I think she's a little scared. She's never seen her gran looking like this and it has obviously upset her. Marie tries to have a brief conversation with her, but she is so tired that she seems to be drifting a little and the conversation lasts little more than a minute.

The district nursing team and palliative care medical team have been regular visitors to the house over recent days, as has the local priest, who is trying his best to offer support and comfort to Claire's dad. It is a very strange feeling being stood in that room. On one hand, I don't want to see such a proud and strong lady struggling and suffering in any way. I wonder whether the best thing would be for her to pass peacefully right now with all her family around her. On the other hand, Claire, Amy and especially Peter are desperately clinging onto every second they have left with her and who on earth would ask for that to come to an end? Every second for them is precious.

I start to feel like a bit of an intruder on the priceless time that Claire should have with her mum, so I go downstairs to get out of the room for a few minutes. Claire follows me down to the kitchen where I make everyone a cup of tea[27]. Claire tells me that Amy was told about her mum's latest devastating scan results just a few hours before she came into Alder Hey and stayed over with Leah to help us out on the 12th of April.

---

27 What could be more quintessentially British? When times get tough, what is the first thing to do? Of course, put the kettle on.

I immediately recall sensing Amy was a little quiet and subdued that night at the hospital. It makes complete sense now. That night must have been excruciating for her and yet again I stand aghast and in awe of the women in this family.

Tuesday 30th April 2019

We have an appointment with Big Bad Barry later today in the hospital. I'm really anxious (more than usual) as I suspect he is going to give feedback from the national sarcoma panel MDT meeting. In truth, I'm absolutely terrified of what that feedback might be. To make matters worse, Claire is unable to join me in the meeting, as she simply does not have the emotional strength to deal with it. I'm going to have to face this one alone.

I arrive at the outpatient clinic at the top of Ward 3B and Barry comes in to meet me in the waiting area. He invites me to follow him to one of the consulting rooms, so I walk slowly behind him as he shuffles along the corridor. My heart is beating out of my chest. I imagine this is how it must have felt walking to the gallows as a condemned man.

We enter the room and I take a seat opposite his desk. There is no conversation between us. I think he can sense my nervousness, but he does little to ease it. The door opens again and Jill from the nursing outreach team comes in to join us. *Oh God!* I think to myself. Barry has called for a chaperone for me. He wouldn't do that if I was about to receive good news, would he? This is not feeling positive at all. Every part of my body just wants to spring up and run out of the room.

Over the course of the next ten minutes or so, Barry then proceeds to tell me, in typical Barry-style, a number of developments. Firstly, the tumour in Leah's body is not particularly responsive to the chemo treatment she has received, which, in his words, 'significantly worsens Leah's prognosis'. I gulp hard, but my throat is dry.

Secondly, he tells me that her case was indeed discussed at the national sarcoma panel on 26th April and the panel agreed two things. I inhale deeply and hold my breath as he speaks. One, that Leah's condition should be officially diagnosed as an undifferentiated sarcoma[28]. Two, that they supported the decision to continue with the use of the VDC-IE treatment protocol for further rounds of chemo. I breathe out a tiny sigh of relief at the latter comment.

Finally, Barry then proceeds to inform me that Leah's case was discussed with the surgical teams from a number of other paediatric oncology centres across England. Namely, Bristol, Sheffield, Manchester and the largest centre in the UK, Great Ormond Street. Every one of them fed back that they didn't feel it was likely that the surgery would be a success and therefore it was probably 'not in Leah's best interests' to operate.

With those few words, he smashed my heart into a million pieces.

---

28 In layman's terms, this means that they have no fucking clue what this is.

Thursday 2nd May 2019

I barely slept a wink last night. While I don't recall Barry actually confirming that the Alder Hey surgeons were not prepared to attempt the surgery, I just cannot see how they possibly can now. How could anyone make a decision to put a child through such high-risk surgery knowing that if the child died on the operating table (as the odds seem to suggest in Leah's case), they would have to live with that for the rest of their life? The surgeons are human beings at the end of the day. Surely it is not possible to just shrug that off. Also, how could anyone make a decision to put a child through such surgery, knowing that the rest of your peers from across the country are telling you not to? If you fail, that would be professional suicide, wouldn't it? I don't know the answers to any of my own questions, but what I do know is that if the surgery is not attempted, Leah has zero chance of survival.

Throughout the last few months, I have desperately clung on to shreds of hope and glimpses of positivity wherever I can find them, but I'm starting to struggle to keep hold of that hope now. In the past, when I've started to doubt, Claire has been there to help me. She has faith. She believes that God can help us, just like her mum does. It is unwavering, and it is powerful, and it has kept her going. Recently more than ever.

Personally, I have always found religion confusing. I've never really felt that a lack of strong belief in a greater power has impacted negatively on my life. Today is honestly the first time I feel that it maybe is. I'm craving that unwavering source of hope now.

I stayed in Leah's room last night as I have for most of this week. I'm terrified that even a single ounce of additional stress on Claire right now will send her over the edge. I cannot possibly share this latest news with her, can I? On top of everything else, it will destroy her.

I would do absolutely anything to be able to talk to her about this latest bombshell, though, and tell her honestly how I feel about it all.

Desperate.

Helpless.

Lost.

I know she would have a way to help me find some hope again. I know it.

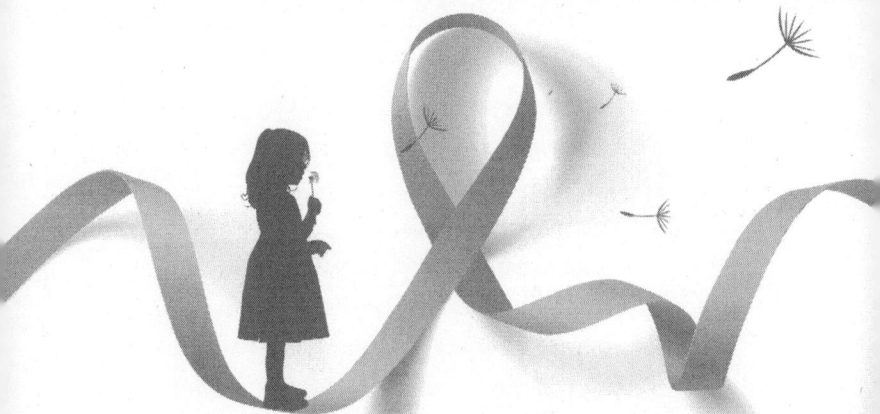

Holding the Bomb

Friday 3rd May 2019

Claire has spent most of the day today at her parent's house, sat by her mum's bedside, along with her dad and sister. They know that time with Marie is rapidly running out and they have made a pact to ensure that they will all be there by her bedside at the very end. The emotional impact of the current situation is enormous on everyone, but the 24/7 bedside presence is also taking its toll physically on Claire and her family. They are all totally drained.

Becky from the Alder Hey oncology outreach team comes round as usual when we're at home to give Leah the GCSF infusion. The drug is administered via a small portable syringe driver that Becky brings with her. The whole thing takes around forty-five minutes from start to finish. Becky sets up the syringe driver, connects it up to

Leah's central line and starts it running. She places it on the arm of the sofa and leaves Leah sat there, watching TV.

She comes into the kitchen to chat to me for ten minutes and I start to make her a cup of coffee. Becky has almost become part of the family over these last few months and when she talks to us about Leah and asks about our family, it is with genuine interest, genuine care and genuine compassion.

While the kettle is boiling, she asks me how Claire's mum is. I just about manage to hold it together as I answer. She then asks me about my sister's wedding and whether Leah is looking forward to going and being a bridesmaid. Leah has obviously been talking to her about it with great excitement over the last few weeks. I pause and stare at the kettle.

The fact is that I have no idea whether Leah will be well enough to go to the wedding in two weeks' time. I have no idea whether Marie will still be with us in two weeks' time. If she is, I have no idea whether Claire will be able to come and watch her daughters as bridesmaids. If she isn't, I have no idea whether Claire will feel strong enough to come. Suddenly, all of these thoughts and the magnitude of the situation starts to overwhelm me once again. I bow my head and break down in tears.

Becky walks across from the other side of the kitchen and gives me a hug. I sit down at the kitchen table while she finishes making the drinks and then she comes and joins me at the table.

'What has happened to your family is just so unfair,' she says to me. 'I wish I had a magic wand because I would use it to make everything right for you all.'

I manage to muster up a smile. She may not be able to make it right, but in a tiny way she has managed to make it a little bit better. I guess that's all she could have done.

Saturday 4th May 2019

Claire went back round to her parent's house just after breakfast. Marie is not really eating anything at all now and she is only able to drink tiny sips of water. She is incredibly weak and just sleeping for long periods of the day. She is also struggling with spells of confusion as a result of the strong pain medication that she is being given to keep her comfortable.

I know how much it hurts Claire to see her mum in this way and she desperately does not want to think of (and worse so, remember) her like this, but she will not leave her bedside for a single second longer than she needs to. Meanwhile, I continue to be at home, diligently keeping on top of Leah's medication and checking her temperature a hundred times a day.

All the time, I feel like I'm holding a ticking time bomb. A time bomb that is getting heavier and heavier by the day. The knowledge that the Alder Hey surgeons have been advised not to attempt surgery on Leah and the fact that Claire doesn't yet know is eating away at me. I cannot tell her, but I worry that, in trying to protect her, I feel as though I'm hiding things from her. This has been going round and round in my head for days now and it is starting to dominate my thoughts.

I settle the girls down for bed at 10pm and then decide

to jump in the shower. As I stand under the warm water, I feel like I can hardly breathe. The anxiety and fear I'm holding is crippling me. The water runs down my face and washes away my tears, but they don't stop flowing. I slump to my knees. My amazing life is dismantling around me and I am completely powerless to do anything about it. I'm holding onto this bomb and it is ticking away in my arms. Tick-tock, tick-tock. It is deafening.

I sit on the floor in the shower for about ten minutes, sobbing uncontrollably. I feel like I am falling apart. I know without a doubt that I have never felt lower in my life. I'm not sure how much more I can take.

Monday 5th May 2019

Marie's condition has continued to deteriorate across the weekend and Claire, Peter and Amy's bedside vigil continues into a third week. Meanwhile, my mental state continues to be on a knife-edge as I battle with understanding how and when to fully update Claire on the current situation with Leah.

I'm sitting watching daytime TV with a cup of tea. It is very early in the afternoon when the day's post drops through the front door. It is the usual bundle of junk mail; a 'not to be missed' broadband offer, a catalogue from a DIY store and a flyer from a local landscape gardening company. In among the mass of wasted paper is a letter from Alder Hey. Within a few days of each and every outpatient consultation at the hospital, we receive a letter summarising the discussion and outcomes from the meeting. Generally, they don't really add any value as they only document everything you were told in the consultation, but I always open them and read them to make sure. Claire, on the other hand, refuses to read them. She detests them as they only serve as a reminder of each hugely painful conversation.

I open the letter. It's from Big Bad Barry. It is a summary of the meeting I had with him on my own last week. I feel the knot in my stomach as I start to read the letter and I try to prepare myself mentally to revisit the conversation that has been on my mind for days.

The content of the letter is mainly just as expected. As usual, I find it hard to read, but it doesn't seem to contain anything new. That is, until I reach the final sentence: '*I did explain to Leah's father that unfortunately I continue to feel her prognosis is poor but of course we will continue to do whatever we can to control Leah's tumour.*'

Whatever we can to '*control Leah's tumour*'.

First of all, I hate that they call it 'Leah's tumour'. It is not hers. She didn't ask for it, she doesn't want it and she sure as hell does not deserve it. But the most disturbing part of that sentence is the use of one single word.

Control.

Not *cure*.

Control.

I don't recall this word being used in the meeting and it's the first time I've ever associated it with Leah's situation. In all previous discussions, Barry has used the word 'cure'. He has always been looking for ways to 'cure' Leah and that word is extremely important to us. That word is positive. It gives us hope. To replace that word with the word 'control' is hugely significant. It is devastating. It suggests they are giving up and accepting defeat. It suggests that the ever-fading light at the end of our tunnel is about to be switched off altogether.

I feel my heart break yet again. We haven't even had a chance to fight her corner and it feels like the towel has already been thrown in. And I still haven't been able to tell Claire.

Tuesday May 7th 2019

Claire came into Leah's room at 1:40am last night to wake me up. She told me that she had received a call from her dad to come to his house. I climbed out of bed and gave her the biggest hug I've ever given in my life. She jumped in her car and I heard her drive away down the road.

I lie awake thinking about her and about her mum for the next hour or so. I stare over at Leah in the bed opposite me. She is sleeping peacefully. I look at her and I smile. Aside from the occasional whirring of her feed pump, the only sound I can hear is Leah's gentle breathing. I think it is the most beautiful sound in the world right now. I can't bear the thought of losing her. I can't think about my life without her. I shed a tear.

I think about life more generally and how small and insignificant I feel. I think about how incredibly precious life is and how unfair it can be sometimes. I think about Marie's promise to Claire… that she would give her own life to save that of her granddaughter. I shed another tear.

At just after 2:30am, I get a phone call from Claire. Marie passed away peacefully ten minutes before Claire arrived at the house. Amy and Peter were at her bedside when it happened. She was just sixty-five years old.

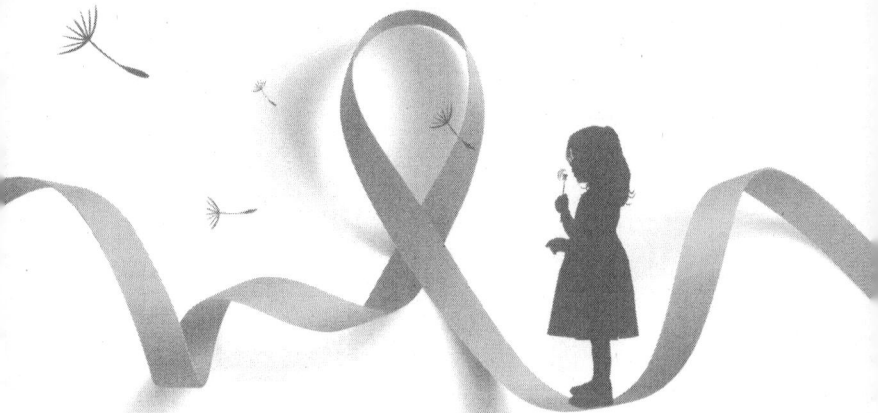

Second-hand Strawberries

Wednesday 8th May 2019

Claire has again left the house early to go and spend time with her dad and sister. She's taken Leah with her. I have barely slept these last few days. There is so much going on in my head. I'm worried about literally everything and everyone close to me right now. I have never been so scared. I still haven't been able to tell Claire the news about Leah's surgery.

Since I arrived home after dropping Phoebe at school at 9am, I've been pacing round the house, rapidly going out of my mind. I feel so anxious. I feel like I can't breathe. I need to talk to somebody. I desperately need somebody to share the weight of this bomb I'm holding. I decide to call my mum.

'Hi, love, are you okay?' she asks.

'No, Mum, I'm not. I'm sorry, but I'm really not. I need to speak to you. Can you come round?'

She agrees to come straight round on her way home from work at midday.

Just after 12:30pm, there is a knock on the front door and my mum lets herself in. I walk into the hall and meet her as she comes through the door. She is holding a small bunch of flowers and some chocolate biscuits. She looks straight at me.

'What's wrong, love? What's happened?' There is a wobble in her voice. I can't answer her. I just throw my arms around her and break down on the spot. She doesn't even have chance to offload the biscuits.

A couple of minutes later, after I've composed myself slightly, we both go into the living room and sit on the sofa. For the next twenty minutes or so, I pour out my heart to her. I tell her about the letter from Big Bad Barry and I tell her they are now only looking to 'control' the tumour. I tell her I haven't been able to update Claire on this information and it is killing me. I tell her how terrified I am.

'You're not on your own with this, son,' she reassures me. 'We're all frightened. She's my granddaughter and I love her, too. We'll all be devastated if she can't survive this, but we'll all support each other and we'll all have to get through whatever is coming together. You need to try and stay strong, love. You need to do that for her. She needs you. Claire needs you. Phoebe needs you. We need to make sure whatever time she has left is as good as it can be and that she knows how much we all love her. You can do this.'

I know my mum doesn't have the answers to any of this,

but she listens and she understands, and she sobs along with me. Just the fact that I've finally been able to share my thoughts makes me feel so much better. Someone else is now holding the bomb alongside me and immediately it feels lighter. However, I'm now conscious that my mum is taking some of the weight and I hope she can share that with others around her if she needs to.

We can do this. We *have* to do this!

Thursday 9th May 2019

Leah should have commenced chemotherapy round six today, but unfortunately her blood levels are not quite at suitable levels again, so we'll have to wait. This is a real concern because the next round of treatment is for six days and Sarah's wedding is in nine days' time. I'm concerned that she might not get to the wedding and I know how devastated she will be if she can't get there.

Claire and her family have started to plan Marie's funeral and this is already becoming a distraction (albeit an unwanted one) from the heartache everyone is now living with every day. It is booked for Monday 20th May, two days after Sarah's wedding. I have no idea whether Claire will be able to go to the wedding either now. In fact, I'll be amazed if she does.

Friday 10th May 2019

Thankfully, Leah's bloods are back up to the required levels and the Alder Hey team have agreed to commence chemo round six today. It is a six-day stay again. I have everything crossed that it will go exactly to plan, and she will be well enough to come home next Thursday and accompany her auntie down the aisle next Saturday.

Claire is coming with us to the hospital for a few hours and then returning home later. She's been really quiet these last couple of days, but she's doing as well as possible considering the circumstances. As Claire, Leah and I leave the house to get into the car, Claire points out the single magpie sat on the lowest branch of the tree in our front garden. It is the seemingly daily symbolic reminder of our misfortune. We both smile ironically at one another.

We drive to the hospital and reach the traffic lights on the filter lane to turn onto the hospital site. Leah is sat in the front seat, so she can tilt it back to take the pressure off her lower back. As we pull up at the lights, she points out that these lights have been on red every single time we have driven up to them. I think about that for a second and I think she's probably right. I can't recall a single time that we've approached them when they've been green, thereby allowing us to drive straight through. Even the traffic lights are seemingly trying to make life that bit more difficult for us now! I'm clearly overthinking everything at the moment. Perhaps just an early sign of insanity?

Tuesday 14th May 2019

Today is day four of six so we're over halfway there. I stayed in with Leah on Friday and last night. My cousin, Emma, did Saturday night to help us out and Claire insisted on doing the overnight stay on Sunday. Leah has been a little up and down over that time. She was sick quite a bit last night, but she had been relatively okay across the weekend.

The last few days have been generally uneventful and we are all familiar with the routine now. However, there was a personal highlight for me earlier on today. Leah woke up in a foul mood and hardly spoke a word to me for a few hours. Lunchtime came round and she point-blank refused to eat anything, which caused another heated exchange of words between us. Eventually, I managed to get her to agree to have a few strawberries from the ward kitchen. She ate two and nibbled on a third one, which she said didn't taste very nice, before she put it back on the plate complete with a side helping of saliva.

Around fifteen minutes later, Big Bad Barry came in to see Leah and check how we both were.

'Ooh, strawberries!' he said as he spotted the plate at the end of the bed. 'I'll have one of those, thank you.'

You can probably guess which one he picked up and put in his mouth. Leah looked at me and smiled widely. It was the only smile I got out of her all day.

Thursday 16th May 2019

After another *long* spell in hospital, Leah's chemo round six finishes today. Claire was in last night and I called her as soon as I woke up at 8am to find out how she was. I'm hoping and praying that Leah is as okay as she can be, and they are happy to let her come home later. Claire tells me that she was okay overnight and her temperature was in the normal range when the nurses did her usual observations this morning. I'm so pleased.

True enough, later in the day, she is given the okay to come home and by late afternoon she is lying on the sofa in our living room in her dressing gown watching TV.

The plan is that the outreach team will be out to give her the GCSF tomorrow as usual. Then, on Saturday, I will take her into the hospital to have her GCSF on the ward early in the morning. All being well, that should leave us enough time to get home, get changed and then drive across to Lincoln for the big day.

In among this, we're obviously worried about whether she'll be well enough on the day and whether we can keep her safe from infection. I'm also worried about Claire and her mental state right now and whether she is capable of going. So far, things are looking positive, but there are a few hurdles to negotiate first.

Oh, and of course there was the usual single magpie on the garden when Claire and Leah arrived home. The universe just doesn't like us to get carried away thinking too many positive thoughts, does it?

Friday 17th May 2019

It is a nurse called Donna from the outreach team who comes out to us to do the GCSF infusion. We've met Donna on the ward once or twice, but this is the first time she's been to our house to see Leah. Donna is quite short with blonde hair and a strong scouse accent. She wears the same purple tunic as the rest of the outreach team.

This uniform has become strangely comforting to me over recent months.

Donna informs me that she's made contact with the main hospital in Lincoln and sent them across a few important details about Leah. This means that they will be prepared if Leah falls unwell and we need to take her in while we are away from home. This is apparently standard practice any time we are planning to be away from Alder Hey. Donna also gives us the contact details for the hospital, so we are as prepared as we can be on our side.

Leah's temperature is stable and she's reasonably well in herself. I message Sarah to let her know that we are still intending to come across in the morning, but we won't know for certain until tomorrow. She sends me back the fingers crossed emoji.

Phoebe has already travelled over to Lincoln with my mum and dad today and she's staying over in a hotel with them so she has time to get ready for the wedding. I spoke to her earlier. She's excited about being a bridesmaid, but she's so worried that Leah might not be there and we might not be there to see her. The fingers crossed emoji is all I can think of right now.

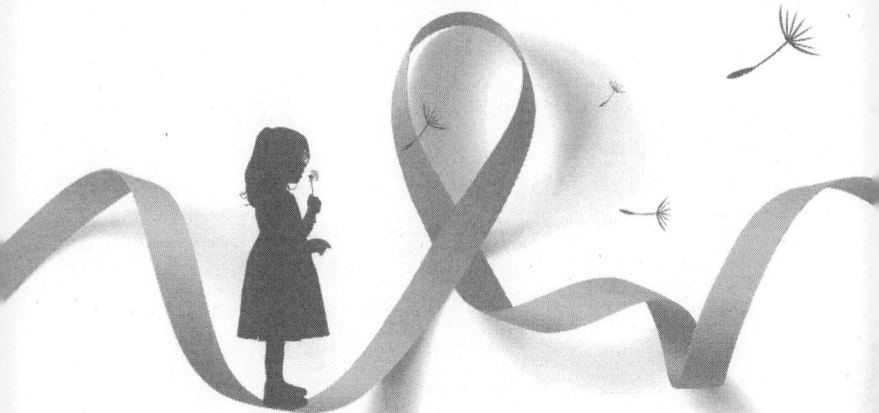

Wedding Bells

Saturday 18th May 2019

The big day has finally arrived. We managed to get through the night without any spiking temperatures. Leah is tired but in good spirits and is bursting with excitement for the wedding. Nothing on this earth is going to stand in the way of her walking down that aisle with her sister and her auntie later on.

The three of us at home get up and dressed early. I drive Leah into Alder Hey for the GCSF first thing, while Claire goes to get her hair done. Despite everything that has happened over this last couple of weeks, she is putting her game face on and she is going to give today a go. In my heart, I'm fairly certain she just wants to spend the day sat in a quiet corner crying, but she knows how important today is for Leah and for Phoebe and for my family, and she's standing up and carrying on. What a woman!

The team on the ward at Alder Hey have been fully prepped that they need to turn everything round as quickly as possible and they are brilliant. We are in and out in double-quick time, return home to collect Claire and then jump in the car. Somehow, the planets seem to be aligning to allow us to go to the wedding.

Before we set off on the two-hour drive to Lincoln, I take a selfie sat behind the wheel of the car with Claire and Leah poking their heads into the background. I post the picture on the #TeamLeah WhatsApp group with the words 'We're on our way' underneath. Immediately, my phone pings with messages from the whole family. They are a mixture of 'Yay' and 'Woop', with one or two smiley face emojis and a couple of crying emojis thrown in the mix, too. I can sense the relief among everyone that Leah is going to make it there for the big day. Right up to this morning, I didn't know myself whether she would or not and it would have absolutely broken her heart if she'd had to miss it.

We arrive at the site of the wedding a little earlier than we expected, at around midday. The site is a beautiful woodland glade with a huge dome tent in the middle. The sun is shining and it feels utterly amazing to have made it here. As we walk onto the site, I spot Phil, my sister's fiancé, over on the far side. In fact, there are only a handful of people milling round the site as we arrive and Phil is one of them. He is checking everything is in place and finishing off the final few tasks[29]. Phil sees us and waves and then makes his way over to see us. As soon as he reaches us, his smile says it all. He gives me a huge bear hug and seems to well up slightly.

'We're so pleased you guys made it. Sarah is absolutely over the moon.'

Half an hour later, Claire has taken Leah off to a small lodge in the corner of the site to get her changed for the big event. While she is away, a large coach pulls into the car park at the edge of the site and the rest of the wedding guests start to filter off. Phoebe jumps off just in front of my mum and dad and sprints over to me and gives me the biggest hug ever. She looks absolutely beautiful in her bridesmaid dress with her hair and nails done. It is so good to see the rest of my family all dressed up and smiling. The feeling of happiness and relief that we have made it across is palpable.

Around ten minutes later, Claire and Leah come back from the lodge. Leah has a matching green bridesmaid dress on and she is now wearing the wig she'd been given from the Little Princess Trust, which has been styled just how she wanted it by our local hairdresser. As soon as I see her coming towards me, I feel that lump in my throat yet again. Seeing her wearing a wig is hard as it is a visual reminder of her struggles, but she just looks so beautiful and so happy and that is all that matters, I suppose.

At 2pm, we are all asked to take our seats in a small

---

29 I would hazard a guess from experience that he's also checked his best man has the wedding rings and been to the toilet at least a hundred times, too.

clearing in the woods, where a large wooden pergola stands in front of rows of fold-out chairs. An aisle made of hessian matting runs through the centre and up to the pergola. We sit down surrounded by the rest of the family on the bride's side. I glance at Phil, who is now stood with his best man at the front. He looks nervous.

Wedding music starts to play and a hush falls over the guests. Everyone turns around to focus their attention on the back of the clearing. Phil's nieces in their bridesmaid's dresses start to shuffle down the aisle. They look really cute and are greeted appropriately by lots of 'Ahhs' from the guests. I notice on the opposite side of the clearing that Phil's sister has a tear in her eye.

Next come my two nephews dressed in little blue tweed suits. They have beaming smiles and are obviously loving being the centre of everyone's attention as they make their way to the front. I catch the eye of my youngest nephew, Cameron, and he smiles at me. I smile back at him.

Next comes the moment I've been waiting for and desperate to see these last few difficult months. Phoebe and Leah, arm in arm, start to make their way down the aisle to the front. They just look perfect... more than perfect. For a moment, I am breathless. I am so proud of them both and what they have overcome to be here today. The emotion is overwhelming and the tears start to flow. Happy tears this time, though.

I glance at Claire linking my arm tightly to my side. She is dabbing tears away with a handkerchief. I am unbelievably proud of her, too, for finding the strength to stand here today, putting the happiness of her daughters before her own personal grief. For that split second, the world is a beautiful place and I feel like the luckiest man on the planet.

I glance around at my mum, my aunties and their families. Everyone is transfixed on the aisle and most are dabbing their cheeks. My older sister then starts to walk down with Sarah's best friend, and following just behind them, the bride herself. My little sis. She looks incredible and so happy. She is beaming and holding my dad's arm tightly as he walks her down the aisle. My dad's eyes are red and puffy; he is clearly struggling to hold the emotions back, too.

I glance to the front of the clearing where Phil is watching Sarah walk towards him. He looks like he is trying hard not to tear up. He turns to look at me and spots my teary face… and he's gone! He starts blubbing like a baby. I'll feel guilty if he has puffy red cheeks on all the wedding photos now. Sorry, not sorry.

The actual wedding ceremony, in keeping with the whole day, is quirky and personal. The person conducting the ceremony is Sarah's friend, Sue, and the whole thing manages to strike the perfect blend of being beautiful, poignant but with a huge dose of fun.

As soon as the ceremony finishes, Sarah and Phil lead a procession of the wedding party back down the aisle accompanied by a brass band, who have magically appeared from the bushes and trees around the clearing. They are playing 'Celebration' by Kool & the Gang. The whole wedding party are now dancing their way across to the main site led by the bride and groom, followed by the band. I can see Leah and Phoebe at the very front of that group, clearly not interested in dancing with their embarrassing Mum and Dad at the back. I can't blame them really. We both look like we've been cutting onions for the last forty-five minutes.

The wedding guests all congregate near to the large dome tent and numerous wine glasses and beer bottles have now appeared in hands. Leah is off posing for photos with the rest of the bridesmaids and the bride and groom. Within about half an hour, she appears back at my side, complaining that her wig is itchy. Seconds later, it is off her head and stuffed into Claire's handbag. The purpose of getting the wig in the first place was because she felt really conscious about people staring at her hair. She was particularly worried about having lots of people do that at the wedding, especially people she didn't know. She must be feeling more confident now and is off buzzing round with her threadbare hair on show to the world. It makes me smile. Thirty minutes later, she returns to ask if she can ditch the bridesmaid dress, too. She changes into a more comfortable party dress and away she goes again to play with her cousins.

Later in the evening, I'm sat with her on my knee at the side of the dance floor and we are talking about the day.

'Have you enjoyed yourself today, darling?' I ask her.

'I've had the best day, Daddy. It's been amazing!'

'Did you like being a bridesmaid then?' I follow up.

'Yes, Daddy, I really liked dancing with Auntie Sarah to the brass band. I think I'd like them to play at my wedding.'

Oh wow. I wasn't expecting that comment. I've tried so hard to hold my shit together all day and then she hits me with that! What is she trying to do to me?

'I really hope they are able to play at your wedding too, baby. I really, really hope so.'

Claire has been quiet all day. I know there are probably a million places she would rather be than here in a field in Lincolnshire, watching everyone smiling and having fun, but she's put her war paint on and she's showed up and that means the world.

Today has been magical from start to finish. The fight may start again tomorrow, but for today, perhaps just for one day, we've had peace on the battlefield. It's hard to describe how much we've needed that.

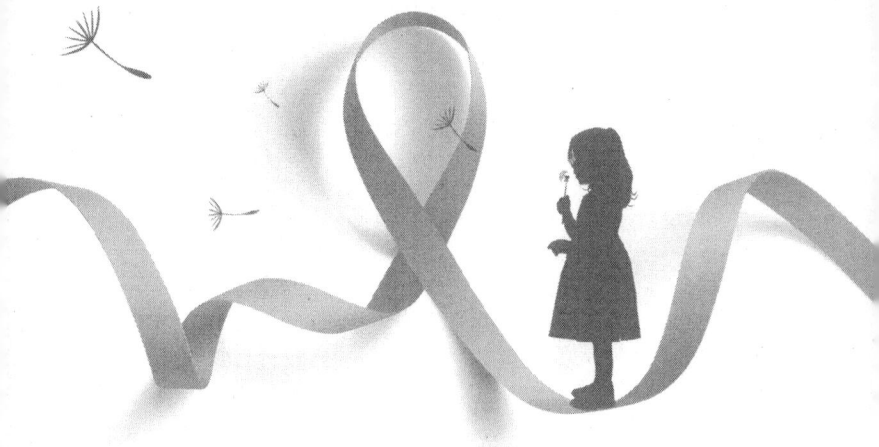

My Wigwam

Claire is my wife of fifteen years and the mother of Phoebe and Leah. Daughter of Peter and Marie, and sister to Rob and Amy. We met when we were just sixteen and worked together at the same local pub/restaurant. We were friends for three or four years before I finally wore her down.

Over the years Claire and I have been together, it has become clear that we share some common values and outlooks on life, but we have very different characters. Claire shares some of her mum's Celtic character traits. She can be fiery and impulsive, but she is passionate and fiercely loyal. On the other hand, I think of myself as quite laid-back, almost passive on occasion. My lack of fire in some situations can really get on Claire's nerves and occasionally prompts an angry reaction (due to fiery Celtic blood). However, I think we generally complement one another fairly well and make it work.

We first got together on New Year's Eve 2001 and after dating for three years, Claire started the conversation about us buying a house together in early 2004. After a bit of 'umming and ahhing', I eventually agreed to look into it. Exactly two days after making that decision, she had calculated our (maximum) budget and booked two different viewings. I had barely had a chance to tap randomly on the walls and check whether there was space for a sizeable shed, when 'our' decision was made. Within three months, we were homeowners.

Our first house was a modest two-bedroom terraced house on a busy road. It was small in size, but it was warm and cosy and it was a fantastic home for us. On Christmas Day 2006, I decided to take the plunge. We were stood in our little dining room when I asked her to close her eyes and I quietly got down on one knee. She opened her eyes and looked down at me, staring back at her all wide-eyed and excited. In all honesty, the look on her face was not quite what I expected or hoped for. It was a look of disappointment. It later turned out that she thought I'd bought her a puppy, therefore seeing me kneeling at her feet was understandably disappointing. However, she did say yes and I think she was happy with that decision. As was I, to be honest, as the engagement ring had saved me a small fortune on a 'big' present for her that year.

In truth, I thought an engagement ring would take a bit of pressure off for a while, but I clearly hadn't learned from the house-buying experience. Within a week, she was buying wedding magazines and visiting wedding fairs. In September 2008, we tied the knot in front of our families and friends. Note to self: a puppy would have been so much cheaper.

In July 2009, we proudly brought Phoebe home from hospital and two became three[30]. Three years later and Leah joined us to make our family complete, albeit our little two-bedroom house was now struggling to cope with the volume of cuddly toys and Disney DVDs.

Perhaps the biggest and most controversial difference between Claire and I relates to how we handle toast. Let me explain…

Claire likes her toast warm and the butter melted on top. Whereas I like mine slightly cooler so the butter sits on the top. In order to achieve the optimum toast temperature, I lean the pieces next to each other to cool down slightly. In a small 'toast wigwam' as Claire describes it in a highly patronising way. The wigwam thing kind of stuck, though, and I often think of it as a metaphor for our relationship over recent years. We are different people with different quirks and different faults and successes. However, we've needed to lean on one another so often over recent times. She's become the equivalent of my toast wigwam. She's prevented me from falling over and helped me to let off steam.

Just for the record, I don't like being covered in butter, so the toast metaphor ends there.

---

30 For the mathematicians among you… yes, she probably was a honeymoon baby!

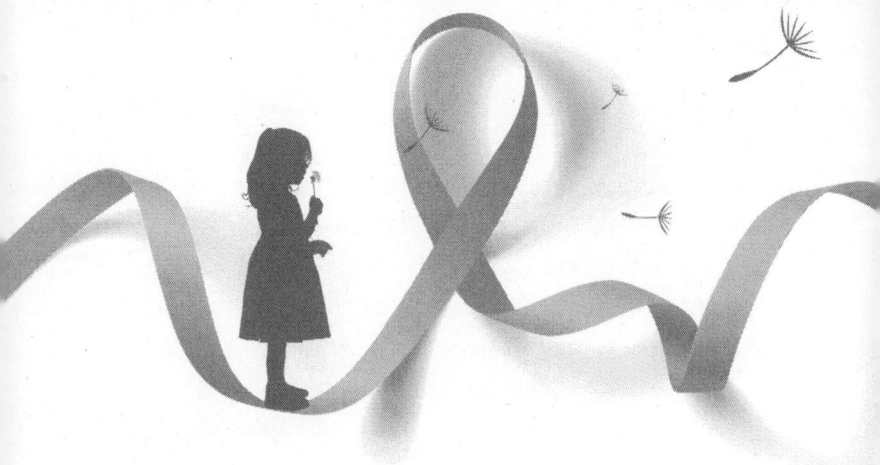

Wild Mountain Thyme

Monday 20th May 2019

Today is the day of Marie's funeral. The day that I think we've all been dreading for the last two weeks. Sarah's wedding has been a positive distraction in a number of ways, but it only ever provided a slight glimmer of light in an otherwise jet-black sky for us. The only positive I can realistically hope for today is that the whole thing passes off well and Claire and the rest of her family can feel like they have done Marie proud.

Marie was a strong feminist and passionately believed that women could do anything that men could do. Claire and her sister, Amy, live by that mantra, too. So much so that they have decided they want to help carry their mum's coffin into the church today. They will do so alongside myself, Peter, Amy's husband, Craig, and Claire and Amy's brother, Rob, who has returned to England from Australia for the funeral.

My mum and dad have agreed to look after Phoebe and Leah during the day and bring them both to a local pub where we have arranged to hold the wake later. Claire has been surprisingly calm and fairly upbeat this morning. It is almost like she is tunnel-vision focused on the day and on ensuring it passes off without any hitches. Claire, Amy, Peter and Rob have planned every aspect with meticulous attention to detail to ensure the day is 'what Mum would have wanted'. Claire, Amy and Marie all shared the same sense of taste in almost everything from clothes to interior decor, so there is absolutely no doubt in my mind that Marie would be happy with everything they have planned.

We drive round to Claire's mum and dad's house late in the morning to meet everyone there. This is where the funeral cortege is to set off from. When we arrive, the house is already full of people. Two of Marie's brothers and a number of their families have travelled down from Scotland this morning to pay their respects.

I walk into the house expecting a sombre mood, but, in fact, everyone is quite chatty and relaxed. It is fantastic to see some of Claire's Scottish relatives, even if the circumstances are not what any of us would have wanted. Even Peter seems to be okay, although I suspect inside he probably just wants to get today out of the way. Everyone is telling Claire stories about her mum when she was younger and they all smile when they describe her. I know in my heart this will mean the world to Claire. I watch her smiling and laughing along with her relatives.

The funeral cars pull up outside the house around half an hour later. We all climb in and make our way behind Marie to the local church. The church is a place that meant so much to Marie in life, so it is only fitting that the building plays a lead role in her final journey.

The cars arrive at the church a few minutes later. There is a large gathering of people outside. Many people I know as friends of the family and ex-colleagues of Marie, but also many people I have never seen before. I notice some of Claire's work colleagues and some of my friends in among the crowd, too. Knowing the support we have around us right now is of great comfort to me, so I can only guess what it must mean to Claire and her family today.

We step out of the cars and gather at the rear of the main funeral hearse. Deep breaths all round. The coffin slides out and the funeral directors help lift it up onto the shoulders of the six of us. We link arms underneath the coffin, take the weight and start to make our way inside the church, led by Claire and Amy, holding their mum with a fierce determination and immense pride.

At the front of the church, we place the coffin onto a stand and a beautiful photo of Marie is placed on a small table next to it. I stare at the photo. I hope she can see how many people have turned up to say goodbye. I think she'd be overwhelmed.

After the priest has said a few words, Claire's brother, Rob, stands up to read the first part of the eulogy to his mum. He seems to struggle a little, but just about gets through it. Next, Amy takes to the altar to say her part. The emotion in her voice is audible throughout, but, again, she manages to get through it. I can feel how important it is to her that she tells the world how she feels about her mum.

Finally, Claire stands up to read her section. I know she's been worried about this and didn't know whether she'd be able to do it. How wrong she was! She stands centre stage in front of the whole church and she speaks clearly and with a passion that I have never heard her speak with in all our years together. Her pride for her mum shines through and she leaves nobody in any doubt as to how much her mum meant to her.

As Claire is talking, my gaze shifts back to the photo of Marie next to the coffin. I think about her words to Claire a few weeks ago. Did she really give up her own fight to save her granddaughter? Is her faith so strong that she has the ability to make a deal like that? What if that is not possible and Leah's fate is already decided? The thought of carrying my daughter's coffin down the same aisle is just unbearable. I feel my mouth dry and a lump in my throat. But what if this is actually true and Marie's personal sacrifice might just hand Leah the lifeline we are desperately searching for? I feel a shiver run down my spine.

I don't know the answers to any of those questions, but as I look at the photo of Marie, I'm certain she would be doing everything she could to fulfil her promise. I feel her strength, her passion and her determination right here, right now in this church. I feel it in the beat of my own heart.

After the church service, a smaller but still sizeable group make their way to the crematorium to say final goodbyes. I have been asked to read a short poem during the ceremony and, when the time comes, I make my way to the front of the room. As I stand at the small lectern, I look out across the faces in front of me. Every one of them full of sorrow with eyes full of tears. I take a deep breath and stare at the poem written on the crumpled piece of paper in front of me. A single teardrop rolls down my cheek and splashes onto the middle of the paper. I wipe my cheek with my right hand and read the poem. Somehow, I manage to struggle through the words. I look up from the lectern as soon as it is over and glance at Claire. Through her tears, she smiles gently at me.

After a few short words from the priest to bring the ceremony to a conclusion, it is time for the final piece of music before we leave the room. Marie never really had a strong love of music, or any particular bands or musicians, so I know it has been difficult for Claire and her family to pick a song that would fit. Eventually, they decided to play the well-known Celtic folk song, 'Wild Mountain Thyme'. The version they picked is a perfect rendition sung by Australian singer Sarah Calderwood. Not only is it a beautiful song, but it nods to Marie's Scottish heritage.

The music starts to play and the room stands in silence as the hauntingly beautiful lyrics float through the air. I am gripping Claire's hand with almost white knuckles and we all have our heads bowed. The emotion is intense, and I can hear the odd sniffle and sob.

As the chorus rouses, I can hear Marie's brothers in the row behind us start to sing the words to the song. Quietly at first, but gradually getting louder. Then, others in the room start to join in. Within a few seconds, half of the room is now in song. It is an intensely powerful moment. It feels electrifying and the goosebumps on my arms prickle. I puff out my chest and burst into song myself. The sense of immense love and support in the room is palpable. A wave of solidarity scooping us all up and raising us high. It is a moment I will never forget, and I can see and feel that Claire and her family all feel exactly the same.

Simply incredible.

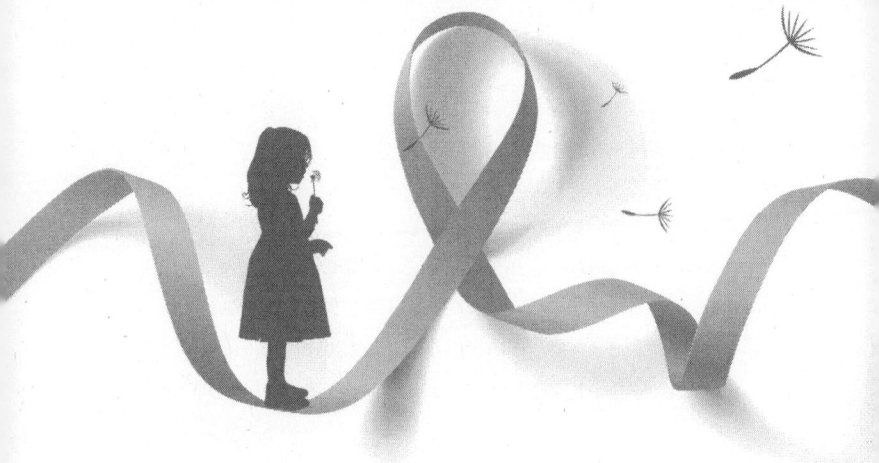

Life's Shit Sometimes

After the service at the crematorium, we go to a local pub for the wake. Claire and her family have pored over the old family albums over recent days to select some photos of Marie to display on a few easels in the corners of the room. Next to one of them is a plate piled high with Tunnock's Tea Cakes and Caramel Wafers for people to sample the delicacies of Marie's hometown. I look through the photos on the easels and there are some of Marie as a child that I've never seen before. I can see the resemblance between Marie in her younger years and Claire. I can also see a similarity with Leah that I've never noticed before. That makes me smile.

Around half an hour later, my mum and dad arrive at the pub with Leah and Phoebe. As soon as I see Leah, I know immediately that something isn't right. She looks upset and she is complaining about stomach pain and struggling to walk properly. My mum tells me she has been fine all day and she has only started to complain about stomach pain in the last half hour or so. I speak to Claire and we decide that she needs to go and get checked out at Alder Hey. Claire obviously cannot leave her own mum's funeral wake, so I agree to take her in. I quickly drive home, get changed out of my black suit and tie, grab the overnight bags (just in case we're staying in) and drive back to the pub to collect Leah before carrying on to the hospital.

We reach the hospital A&E half an hour later and the department is really busy. The queue for reception is out of the main doors. This means two things for us. One, it might take a while for Leah to get seen. Two, there are an awful lot of people in this space, including a lot of poorly looking children. Leah's condition and the vulnerabilities that it creates for her always makes me nervous taking her anywhere where there is a crowd, but when half of the crowd are snot-filled children, coughing and spluttering over their parents' shoulders, I am beyond anxious.

After around twenty minutes of queuing and simultaneously trying to keep a safe distance from everyone else in the room, we eventually reach the front of the front. I give our details to the lady behind the desk and we are promptly shepherded into the room behind the reception while we wait to be seen. It is around 6pm. Leah is really tired and her stomach pain just does not seem to be subsiding. I'm worried about her. I mean, I'm *always* worried about her, but, right now, I'm even more worried than usual.

After an hour of waiting, one of the nurses comes in to see Leah and does the usual checks. Soon after that, we are taken through into one of the cubicles in the main department.

I glance at my watch. It is 8:27pm. Leah is lying on the trolley in the cubicle and I'm sat on a plastic chair next to her. She is visibly uncomfortable and her stomach pain seems to be worsening. So is my anxiety. An hour or so later, after a couple of fleeting visits by the nurses and a junior doctor, she is eventually seen by the consultant on duty.

The consultant is a female with short dark hair and a slight Irish accent. She looks quite tired, but I'm not entirely surprised given the number of people in the waiting area outside. After talking to Leah and I for five minutes and having a good feel of Leah's abdomen, she decides to send us down to the radiology department for an X-ray. When we return around thirty minutes later, the decision is made to put Leah onto a PCA[31] to help her manage the pain as things just don't seem to be getting better for her.

It seems to take forever to get the equipment set up and working, but once the pain medication kicks in, Leah finally seems to settle and almost instantly falls asleep. It is now 11:06pm. With Leah now peaceful, I feel like I can breathe for the first time all day. Within a couple of minutes, I fall asleep with my head on the trolley next to her.

---

31 Patient-controlled analgesia: a machine that administers pain relief based upon the patient pressing a button.

At around 11:30pm, I am woken by the same consultant. She informs me that the X-ray from earlier shows nothing out of the ordinary. Therefore, she believes Leah's stomach pain is directly related to the sarcoma. I close my eyes, bow my head and give a small ironic chuckle as if to say, 'Of course it is! As if today could not get any worse!' I appreciate that I am completely shattered both physically and mentally, but, even so, her words still cut through me. They really hurt. This is all starting to feel inevitable now. It feels like she's losing her fight.

The A&E team have decided to keep Leah in the hospital overnight and the plan is that she will be reviewed by the oncology team in the morning. Unfortunately, there are no beds available on Ward 3B and so we need to wait for a bed to become available elsewhere.

At 1:30am, one of the ED nurses comes into the cubicle and wakes me up to tell me there is now a bed available for Leah on ward 4A. Leah is fast asleep and looks peaceful. I gather up our bags and sit patiently waiting to go up to our new home for the night. I am exhausted. Twenty or so minutes later, the consultant pops back into the cubicle to tell us the porter is coming to take us up to 4A.

'Do you know we buried Leah's gran today... my mother-in-law?' I say to her. I'm not actually sure what I wanted to achieve with the comment. I think I just want someone to appreciate how hard today has been. Perhaps it is a slight cry for help?

She looks at me open-mouthed. I can see the compassion in her eyes as they soften. She doesn't have the words to respond, so she just walks across the cubicle and gives me a hug. It is one of those hugs that say more than words ever can. I don't really have the strength to hug her back.

The porter comes in to push Leah's trolley up to 4A and, just as we're leaving the cubicle, the consultant says to me, 'I'm really sorry you're going through this. Life can be really shit sometimes, can't it?'

'It certainly can,' I reply.

Head bowed, shoulders slumped forward, with several bags hung over them, I follow Leah's trolley out onto the corridor and up to 4A.

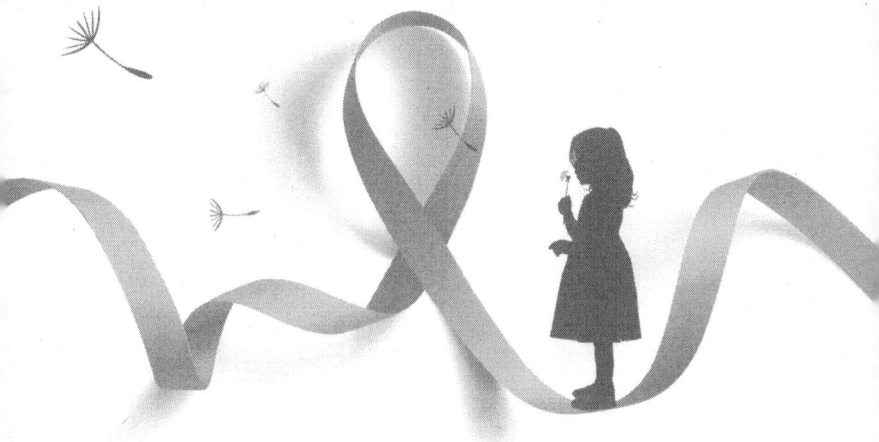

Somebody You Love

On the long list of shitty days that I've had over recent months, yesterday was definitely up near the top of the pile. Just to put the icing on the cake, when we arrived on ward 4A just before 2am, there was only one solitary pillow to be found anywhere in the room. I placed that under Leah's head and spent the night on the small sofa, fully clothed, under a thin blanket, resting my head on my trainers. It's fair to say I didn't sleep too well and I've woken up this morning feeling flat and a little defeated, if I'm honest.

Leah's stomach pain was managed well overnight thanks to the PCA and she's woken up feeling seemingly much better this morning. I've been watching her for the last hour or so and she hasn't pressed the PCA button once, which suggests a significant improvement from where she was last night.

Just before lunchtime, Big Bad Barry comes over to the ward with his Big Bad Entourage of junior doctors and senior oncology nurses and reviews Leah. He feels her stomach and asks her a handful of routine questions. He turns to face the other members of his 'Big Bad gang' and discusses a few things with them. Then, he promptly turns back to me. I'm braced for impact.

He concludes that Leah's stomach pain is actually completely unrelated to the sarcoma. Given that she seems to be managing okay without the need for the PCA now, he requests that she is taken off it and then tells me I can take her home later that day. I had more or less spent the whole of last night terrified that we were starting to see the signs of a real deterioration in Leah's condition. Therefore, this morning's news is quite a turnaround and a very pleasant surprise. I pause for a second to take the good news in. It is possibly the first bit of genuine positive news about Leah's condition that I've heard in over three months. I mean, it's far from amazing – let's be clear about that – but at least it is not just another descent into the abyss.

Barry being Barry obviously won't let us get away on a relative high note. He expresses his great concern again at the lack of chemotherapy response from Leah and reiterates the surgical challenge that this presents. *Like I don't already know this? Please just let us go home, Barry. We've had quite enough bad news already, thank you!* His words make me think again about the surgical challenge that may lie ahead for Leah. I just want to scream at him, *'Just do it!'*

This is ironic, really, given that I'm fairly sure I still have the shape of the Nike tick imprinted on my left cheek from last night's makeshift pillow.

Tuesday 28th May 2019

It's scan day today. The next hugely significant milestone for us all. I hate seeing Leah's little face peering out of the hole in the MRI machine. It never fails to make me upset looking at her as I reflect on her journey so far. Claire always sits in the chair next to me and spends the duration of the scan time praying. She is obviously being far more productive and proactive than me in that respect.

We'll find out soon enough whether Leah's body has had a delayed response to the chemo or not. If she hasn't, I dread to think what that means. I can't let myself get into that headspace because it paralyses me every time. We continue to hope for a positive outcome and hope Marie is up there pestering the life out of the Big Guy Upstairs to help us out.

Thursday 30th May 2019

Leah is scheduled to start the seventh round of her chemo treatment today. However, Barry has told us that no decision will be made about ongoing treatment until her case has been discussed at the next national sarcoma panel meeting. The next meeting of the panel is tomorrow, so we have no choice but to wait and hope and pray that they believe further treatment is worthwhile based on the latest scan images being positive.

Again, it feels like Leah's fate rests in the hands of a group of people who have never met her or us, and we have absolutely no say in the matter. Their decision could determine the course of the lives of the whole of my family and yet we are powerless to influence it. It is excruciating. Nonetheless, we cling onto hope wherever we can find it. Incredibly, we have put all our trust in Marie now. The one person who isn't actually here with us is possibly the only person who can really turn this around for us all.

Monday 3rd June 2019

After a(nother) weekend of trying and failing to distract ourselves from the latest pending decision around Leah's treatment, Monday arrives. We have an appointment with Big Bad Barry later this afternoon and I anticipate that we will hear her fate – both in terms of the MRI scan results and the outcome of the sarcoma panel discussion.

I'm incredibly anxious. My fingernails look like chewed husks of corn on the cob. I'm trying not to let it show to others, especially Claire and Leah. We've decided not to take Leah to the appointment. There is a high probability that we will be told more difficult news and we are aware that we might need time to process the information and decide how best to communicate it to her.

Despite every bone in her body not wanting to sit in front of Barry and hear him tell us anything that might be more bad news, Claire has agreed to accompany me to the appointment. She insists on coming as she doesn't want me to deal with this on my own. I have mixed feelings about this. Yes, I don't want to have to sit through even more (possibly the worst) bad news alone, but I also don't have the strength to pick Claire up if she hits the floor. I'm barely able to keep myself going at the moment.

We arrive at the clinic on time and take a seat in the busy waiting room. Ten minutes later, Barry appears at the door. He says goodbye to the family he has just seen before us and then comes to greet us. He beckons us to follow him and yet again we walk the 'walk of doom' down to the clinic room at the front of the ward. Nobody says a word. My heart is racing. I'm gripping Claire's hand tightly.

Inside the clinic room, Barry starts by giving us the results of the scan from Tuesday. The measurements taken from the scan suggest that the overall size of the tumour has reduced by around a centimetre in all dimensions. The tumour has finally started to respond in a small way to the treatment! I breathe out a huge breath. It is audible.

My initial reaction is that this is incredible news. Perhaps the reduction is not as significant as we had all hoped, but, at last, this is finally some positive news. At last, there is a reaction to all this horrible treatment she's had to go through. Marie is doing it! She's bloody doing it for Leah! I glance across at Claire. Her eyes are looking upwards and she has a tear in the corner of her eye.

Before we can get too carried away, though, Barry continues. While there has now undoubtedly been a response to the chemotherapy, it is a very minor response.

It is not of the magnitude that we wanted and, in fact, *needed* to see. Essentially, Barry tells us that he is unsure about the possible value in continuing with the current chemotherapy protocol. Oh God, no!

He continues by telling us that there was a discussion among the panel on Friday about whether to switch to a 'second line' chemo as an alternative. He tells us that he remains undecided on this issue and will speak again to Prof. Bannan in Manchester to get another view. Given the relatively poor response Leah has had to the first line chemo treatment, Barry doesn't expect that she would have any more of a response to second-choice treatments. While he stops short of ruling out further treatment, I'm in no doubt as to where his thinking is at present. I think Barry sensed that we were reading his body language and the words he wasn't saying, and our resultant unease.

In typical Barry-style, he tries to placate us with some reassurance. 'I have to say that Alder Hey has an excellent Palliative Care team.'

Not what we needed to hear! This more or less confirms where his thinking is. Claire is still looking to the ceiling.

I start to feel that haze descending in my head and Barry's words are becoming more and more distant and echoey. I'm getting that out-of-body experience again, which I've felt before in this situation.

He effectively then reiterates the conversation that he and I had a few weeks earlier. He mentions the view of the surgical team that operating was 'unlikely to be in Leah's best interests'. This time, Claire is obviously in the room. I can see the information we are being given is physically difficult for her to hear, but she remains silent, processing what she is hearing. I wonder if her mum is here alongside her, helping her to make sense of everything.

'Do you have any questions?' Barry asks.

I sit in silence, staring at the wall above his head. Claire looks him straight in the eyes and starts to talk.

'Have you ever had to sit next to somebody you love and watch them pass away, Barry?' She is completely calm and controlled. Her words delivered with precision and thought.

Barry squirms a little in his seat. He is visibly taken back by the question. He stumbles over his words slightly but eventually replies, 'No, I haven't personally, but I would imagine some of the members of the MDT have had that experience.'

Claire then responds, 'So, *no* is the answer, Barry. You haven't ever had to do that? Well, I have. Three weeks ago. Let me tell you that it is hard. Really hard. The hardest thing imaginable. What you are telling me is that you and the rest of this group are making a decision not to operate on our daughter? Not to even give her a chance? We are the people who will have to live with the consequences of that decision. I know exactly what those consequences are and they are completely devastating. Yet you are all seemingly making that decision without even discussing this with us, her parents, the people who have to deal with what that decision actually means. I sat through hell. For days. No, actually for weeks. Nursing my mum in her final days due to this disease and eventually having to say goodbye to someone I love. Now you are sat here, telling me that I will have to go through all that again with my daughter?'

The room is silent. The hairs on the back of my neck are standing up. Barry simply doesn't know what to say. He pauses for a moment, before responding, 'I hear clearly what you are saying, and I will take that back to the MDT group. As I've said, the big decision here is a decision around surgery. I am not a surgeon, so I cannot make that decision, but what I can do is ask the surgeons to meet you themselves so you can have this conversation with them. I must manage your expectations here, though; the absolute best they are likely to offer you is the possibility of agreeing to open Leah up and have a look at what they can possibly do. They certainly won't give you any guarantees, though.'

'We understand that, Barry' I jump in and reply. 'We would be grateful if you could arrange for us to see the surgeons as soon as possible so we can understand more about where things are. It is important for us to have a voice in this conversation and any decision being made. All we are asking, Barry, is that you don't give up on our daughter because, I promise you, we won't.'

'I won't give up, believe me,' Barry replies. 'I will ask whether the surgeons will agree to meet you and come back to you.'

'Thank you,' says Claire.

I can almost feel the crackle of electricity in my body as we leave the room.

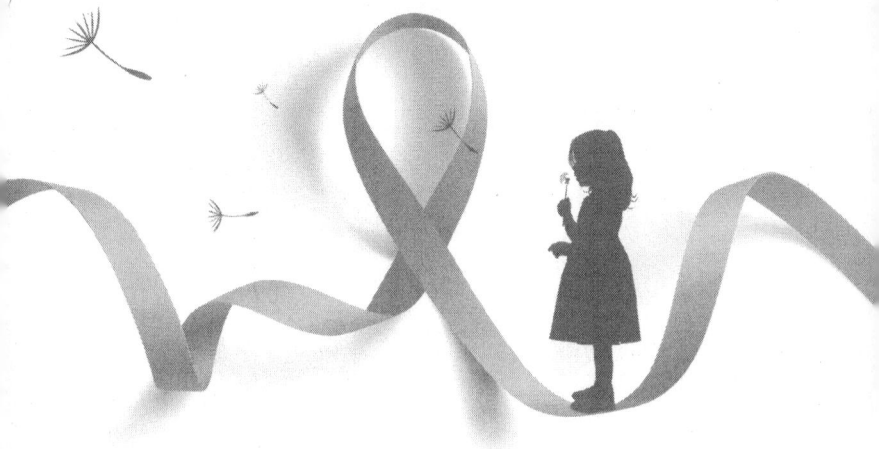

Losing My Religion

Driving home from the hospital alone was often the time I started to think deeply about all of the things happening in my life. On occasion, my mind would drift onto the subject of religion. I mean, surely, *surely* if there is a God up there and He/She/It is truly a force of good and of kindness and compassion, why on Earth would they allow Leah to become so poorly? She is a young child with a huge heart, and she has more natural kindness and compassion than most adults I know. Why, oh why, would any God *not* want people like her on this planet? I don't understand. This thought was often one that I would battle with and one that would often make me really angry – even though I had no idea who to be angry with.

One afternoon in early June, while Claire is on the day shift in the hospital, her dad comes round to our house to drop Phoebe off. It is really good to see him, although

I think it is fair to say he doesn't look himself. He is pale and a little distant when I speak to him. Completely understandable given the circumstances, but still not nice to see him looking like that. He is probably looking at me thinking the exact same thing, though.

Before he leaves, we chat in the kitchen and he tells me that he wants to help us more. Marie has now gone and he is obviously broken-hearted, but he wants to help in any way he can. He acknowledges that he can't bring Marie back, but he wants to do anything and everything he can to ensure we don't lose Leah, too. He mentions Marie's words about letting her go in order to save Leah. She obviously said the same to him as she said to Claire. He gets emotional as he says it. I find his strength remarkable and I thank him. I only wish there *is* something he can do to help. He asks me how Claire is doing.

'As well as she can, Peter,' I reply. 'She's doing incredibly well considering the circumstances.'

There is, however, one issue that I know she is really struggling with, and it is one that I don't feel I can help her with.

'Actually, Peter, there is something you can help me with…' I say.

I start to talk to him about religion. More specifically, about Claire and religion. I tell him that I am really worried about her and the fact that she seems to be all over the place with respect to her faith. She is really angry a lot of the time and has genuinely started to question her faith. For the first real time in her life, she seems to be wondering whether there is someone listening to her prayers. None of the world makes sense to her and she is terrified.

My worry is that if she loses her faith, then she also loses a huge part of what she is as a person. I have tried to speak to her about it and advise her not to give up. There is so much uncertainty about the future that it is impossible to predict what will happen, or whether her many prayers will eventually be answered. I know one hundred per cent that I am not the right person to speak to her about this, though. Therefore, I am asking Peter whether he can help. Perhaps he could chat to her and help her to try and make sense of this whole mess in some way?

Peter says that he understands the situation and he will try his best to help her. He then proceeds to tell me that he, too, is struggling with his own faith. Of course he is! How ignorant of me to think he wouldn't be battling with those same issues himself. I have no idea what is real and what isn't, but I do know that if there is anyone on the other end of Claire and Peter's prayers, now is the time for them to provide a response.

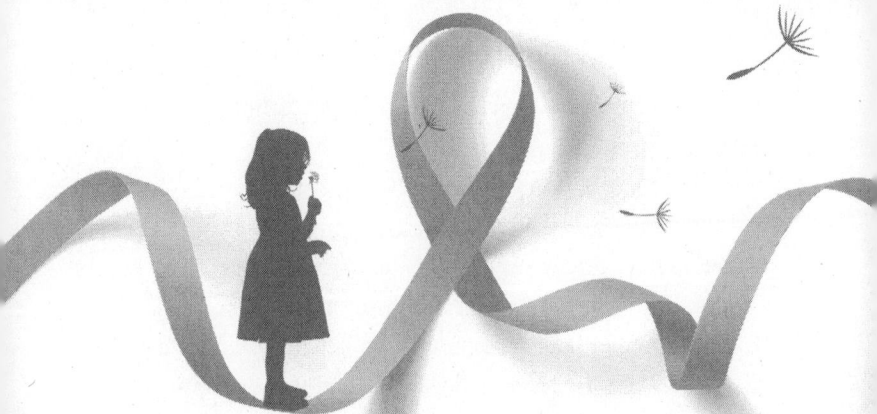

Good Luck, Jaxon

Tuesday 4th June 2019

I am awoken from a very deep sleep just after 8am this morning by the sound of my phone ringing at the side of the bed. Bleary-eyed and with a gruff voice, I answer the call.

'Hello?' I grunt.

'Hello, Barry Pilling here' is the response.

Immediately, I'm on high-alert and my heart rate increases. Barry confirms that he has asked the Alder Hey surgical team to meet with us and discuss the situation with Leah. He tells me that he will come back to us to confirm if a meeting will go ahead and, if so, when. I thank him and I take the opportunity to ask him what it means to us if the surgeons refuse to attempt the surgery. Claire and I have been talking about this a lot over recent days. If we get a negative response from the surgical team at Alder Hey, what else can we do? We can't just give up on her. What might plan B look like?

Barry tells me that there is a world-leading cancer hospital called Memorial Sloane Kettering (MSK) in New York in America. He informs me that he has a contact in the surgical team over there and it might be a possibility to take Leah across to the US as an alternative way forward.

This is an interesting comment and is something Claire and I have not given much thought to previously. He agrees to open dialogue with the surgeons at MSK to gauge their opinion on whether they felt the tumour in Leah's body was operable or not. This could prove to be crucial in terms of giving us another option if the answer from the Alder Hey surgeons is ultimately a no. Another tiny glimmer of hope, perhaps?

Wednesday 5th June 2019

Barry calls again, randomly and out of the blue as usual, putting the fear of God in me once more. He told me that he had spoken to Professor Bannan in Manchester again and, following her advice, he has now decided that Leah should receive the next three rounds of chemotherapy after all. The basis of the decision is simply the fact that the results of the last three rounds of treatment show that the tumour is responding, albeit slowly. Therefore, three more rounds may well give a further, and perhaps more significant, reduction.

This is such a huge relief. As far as Claire and I are

concerned, if the treatment is demonstrably having a positive impact, even just a small one, at least it is stopping the bloody thing from growing – therefore *it is working, so why the hell would you stop it?*

Barry goes on to confirm that Leah's bloods from the last blood sample are back within the safe range and therefore he would like her to come into hospital to commence chemo round seven tomorrow.

Thursday 6th June 2019

We arrive at Alder Hey at 10am on the dot, as requested. This round of treatment will be the three-day stay. The three-day stints have proven to be far less challenging for us to manage as a family, providing, of course, that Leah is not too ill from the drugs. I'm planning to cover tonight in the hospital; my cousin, Emma, is doing tomorrow night; and Claire wants to stay with her on Saturday, so that's our plan for the next few days.

Leah has been allocated room four for the next three days, which is about halfway down the ward corridor just past the main nurse's station. As we make our way up to the room, carrying multiple bags and pushing Leah in her wheelchair, we walk past room three. This is the room that Tom, Suzie and Jaxon have been staying in for the last six months or so. I notice that some of the posters and drawings that have always been stuck on the glass doors of the room have been taken down. My heart sinks at this and I shudder at the thought of what might have happened.

We go into room four and unpack all our things. Leah

settles onto the bed and immediately flicks on the TV to watch a cartoon. I make my way to the parent's kitchen to put some milk in the fridge and I pass Tom on the corridor. He smiles and says hello. He certainly doesn't look distraught. I ask him if everything is okay. He informs me that Jaxon has been given a place on a clinical trial in Manchester starting next week, so, after almost twelve months stuck on this ward, they are finally getting ready to leave.

I can't help wishing they were leaving under more certain and positive circumstances, but it was Tom that told me back in February about how important it has been to them to maintain hope. This clinical trial will offer them hope and therefore it is a positive situation for them. Around an hour later, I watch the three of them saying their goodbyes to the ward staff and heading off down the corridor.

Over recent months, I've found Tom's words to be really powerful and helpful. Hope is just so important. It is one of the only things that has given us the strength to continue. I have hope in my heart for Jaxon, Tom and Suzie now, too.

Friday 7th June 2019

Leah had an up-and-down night last night. We had a few hours between 2am and 3am when her oxygen levels dropped and I was awoken by a doctor coming into the room to review her. At one point in the early hours, the ward nurses were asking Leah to put an oxygen mask on as they were so concerned. She was having absolutely none of it! Even at 3am, she is feisty and determined. If she doesn't want to do something, good luck to anyone who is trying to get her to do it. As much as I think she's incredible, I could equally throttle her sometimes.

We both wake up late in the morning due to being disturbed during the night and, despite getting a small lie-in, we are both really tired this morning. I've agreed with Claire that I will cover the whole day today until Emma comes in later to take over from me to give her a day off. This is going to be a long day.

Leah seems to be a little 'chesty' and full of cold since she woke up, so it's probably not too surprising that her oxygen levels are not where they need to be. I woke up to see the oxygen mask and the tubing trailing on the floor at the side of the bed. I guess, in the end, the nurses must have accepted defeat.

Leah sleeps on and off for most of the day and isn't hugely chatty when awake. She's well and truly fed up with all this now. She's not the only one. Emma comes onto the ward at around 7pm and tags me out. I make sure she has everything she needs and that Leah is okay before I leave for the night. Leah has perked right up in the last hour or two (she's probably just had enough sleep now) and Emma shows me a bag she has brought in that contains a pamper kit and face gems. Something tells me Leah isn't going to sleep any time soon.

Sunday 9th June 2019

Chemotherapy round seven finishes today and Claire will be bringing Leah home later to recover. She called me earlier to tell me she had spoken to Barry. He is the consultant on duty this weekend and they had a conversation when he came to see Leah as part of the ward round this morning.

The latest news is that we have an appointment with the Alder Hey surgical team at 10am on Wednesday. My heart is pounding at the thought. Have they already made the decision not to operate and this meeting is just a tick-box exercise? Are they genuinely undecided and giving us a chance to help them make the decision? Have the surgeons at MSK in America agreed to try the surgery and are going to tell us we need to remortgage our home to pay for it?

We'll find out on Wednesday, but one thing is for certain: we've at least jumped the first hurdle simply by the fact that they've agreed to talk to us. For that, I'm really grateful already.

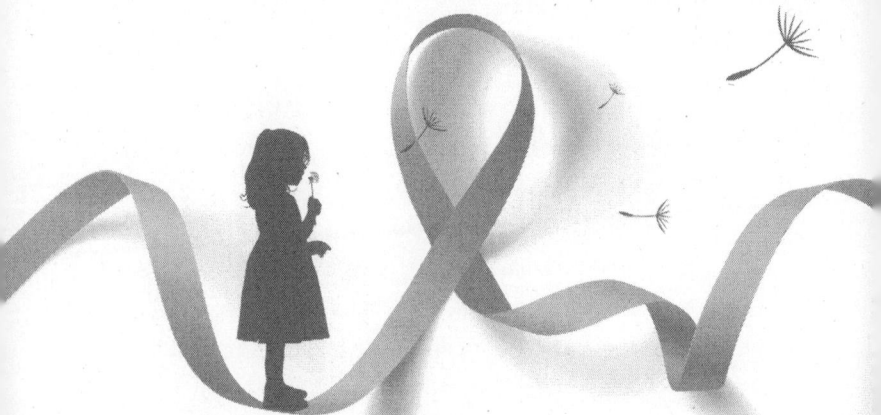

The Firing Squad

Wednesday 12th June 2019

I wake up just after 5am with a million and one questions flying around in my head again. This has sadly become a fairly normal situation for me, but this morning it feels different. It is a strange mix of fear, excitement, anxiety and hope all mixed into one. I genuinely have no idea what the surgeons are going to say to us today, but at least now we have a chance to give them our views and to share our hopes and fears. At least today we get to be part of the most important discussion of our lives and that is all we've been asking for these last few weeks.

Peter comes round to the house at 8am to sit with Leah. She has been given all her meds and her feed and she is asleep in bed. He kisses Claire and Phoebe as we leave the house just after 8:30am and wishes us all well.

We drop Phoebe off at school on the way and both kiss her slightly more than usual before she runs off into school. Then, we make our way to Alder Hey.

Claire and I arrive at the outpatient department at around 9:30am. We sit in silence, gripping each other's hand tightly. In my other hand, I have a small notepad on which I have scribbled down a list of questions to ask and points to raise with the surgeons. The outside of the notepad is glistening slightly from the sweat of my palm.

Just before 10am, one of the clinic room doors opens and out walks Barry. He has clearly been part of a pre-meet with the surgeons. They obviously now have their position aligned and agreed. We just have to wait a few more agonising minutes for it to be delivered to us. Our expectation is that we will be told that surgery for Leah is not going to be an option. Claire and I have discussed this exact scenario for many weeks, so I know we are both completely of the same opinion. We know how difficult this situation is and we are well aware of what the other hospitals across the country have said. However, we are in agreement that we need to push them to try. We have to know with all our hearts that we have given her every chance of survival. Somehow, we both feel that if they give her a chance, she will take it. Marie told Claire that she had given up her own fight to try and save her granddaughter, and she has never, and would never, let her down. They just have to give her a chance.

Around ten minutes after Barry has left the room, the door opens once more and out walks one of the surgeons. I immediately recognise her. Her name is Joanne Minford.

I have met her on a few occasions during my time working at Alder Hey. I have no idea whether she will remember me or not, though. It feels strangely uncomfortable knowing that I know her – I'm not sure whether that goes in our favour or not. I'm pretty sure I bought her a coffee on one occasion when we met, although I do accept that agreeing to undertake potentially career-ending surgery on my daughter is probably not a reasonable payback.

Ms Minford comes across to collect us from the waiting room. She smiles and introduces herself, shaking both Claire and my hand in turn. She gestures towards the clinic room to ask us to make our way in. On the walk to the room, she looks at me.

'I know you, don't I?' she asks.

'Yes. Hi, Jo,' I reply. I'm trying to read her body language and she looks nervous. This makes me more nervous.

Jo shows us into the room where two people are sat on two of three chairs lined up next to the far wall. They both stand as we enter the room and smile and shake our hands as we walk in. We take our seats on the two chairs lined up opposite them. The two others in the room quickly introduce themselves as Mr Matthew Jones and Ms Fiona Murphy. They are two other members of the surgical team.

Jo starts the conversation. 'Firstly, can I say on behalf of us all how sorry we are that you find yourselves in this situation and rest assured we will do everything we possibly can to help your daughter.'

Immediately, I feel uplifted by this statement. We are desperate for them to do everything they possibly can, but the operative word is 'possible'… *what is actually possible*?

Jo then continues with a question that catches me off guard slightly. 'Before we get into the conversation, is it possible to see a photo of Leah?'

It dawns on me immediately that they have never met her. They must have pored over numerous scans of her abdomen, and they probably understand the inner workings of many of her main organs in detail, but they have never actually seen her face. They have never seen the beautiful, inspiring, kind-hearted and courageous little girl that we know and love. My brain is working overtime to understand this. Why would they want to see Leah's face if they have no intention of even attempting the surgery? Surely that would just be cruel to us.

My heart races faster as I fumble for my phone in my pocket. I flick it on, navigate to my camera roll and scroll to a picture of Leah I took at home earlier this week. She is stood in her bedroom, holding Harry the hamster with a huge smile on her face. I hand the phone to Jo.

'Thank you. She's beautiful,' says Jo and shows the picture to Matthew and Fiona.

'Yes, she is,' says Claire. 'She's really special.' She smiles at the three surgeons.

Over the next twenty minutes, the surgical team proceed to explain what would be required in terms of the surgical procedure. They start to describe to us in detail the complexity of the operation. After a couple of minutes, Jo reaches back and picks up a large object from the desk behind her. It is coloured bright yellow and bright pink and looks like some kind of plastic model. It is difficult to make out exactly what it is, but then Jo begins to explain.

She holds the model in her right hand and starts to point at the various different parts, explaining what each of them are. The pink parts are Leah's main arteries and veins at the bottom of her abdomen; the white parts represent the urethral stents that Leah had inserted earlier in the year; and the large yellow part in the centre, encasing everything, is the tumour. It is huge and it is ugly and I bow my head for a second when Jo explains what it is.

While I was aware of the approximate size of the tumour from previous discussions with Barry and some of the letters we'd received, staring at it in front of my eyes is something else entirely. It seems larger than I imagined in my head. It is horrifying.

Jo then hands the model to me and I take hold of it. It renders me speechless. How on earth does something this big exist inside my daughter's body? I'm now holding in my hands the very thing that is gradually killing my precious little girl. It is quite a chilling experience. I can only imagine it might feel similar to a parent coming face to face in court with someone accused of murdering or seriously injuring their child. The evil culprit finally unmasked before my eyes. So this is what you really look like? I'm not sure I can accurately describe my hatred for you.

At the same time, I am very aware that the team would not have gone to the lengths of creating this model if they had already made the decision not to attempt the operation. Why would they bother if they weren't considering it? I have a strange mix of both extremely positive and extremely negative emotions going through me simultaneously. I offer the model to Claire, but she refuses to take it from me. She cannot bear to look at it, so there is no chance that she is going to hold it.

The surgeons then begin to explain the specific risks of the surgery. The conversation becomes a little hazy and a little overwhelming at this stage, but essentially Matthew describes the following to us:

1. It is impossible for them to know at this point whether it is possible to attempt to remove the tumour. They will only truly know if it is possible if they open Leah up and go into her abdomen.
2. The chances of the tumour being operable have been estimated at just twenty per cent.
3. There is a serious risk of life-threatening blood loss from the procedure and this could cause Leah to die on the operating table.
4. Should the tumour turn out to be operable, the task of removing it is extremely delicate due to the location of Leah's major blood vessels in relation to the tumour. The surgeons have estimated that there would be around a fifty per cent chance of Leah losing the use of her legs or dying post-operatively from complications relating to blood flow to her lower body.

In my head, I'm busy working out the maths. I calculate that probably leaves us with around a ten per cent chance of the procedure being successful and leaving Leah alive and with the full use of her legs. Ten per cent. I'm not sure how I feel about that.

Jo then continues and summarises the position of the surgical team. 'We have obviously discussed Leah's case in detail, and we have discussed it with a number of other colleagues. Our biggest concern is that we attempt the procedure and we risk stealing perhaps six months of time that you might have with Leah.'

Boom. There it is. I've steered well clear of asking the 'How long has she got?' question since day one and so has Claire. The truth is, it is a negative question and I'm not actually sure it helps either of us in any way to know the answer. However, we now know the answer whether we wanted it or not. Six months is obviously all they believe she might have. I speak first in response to Jo's comment.

'The truth is, Jo, that we feel we've already lost Leah to an extent. Six months ago, she was playing football and running round with her friends. Now, she can barely get round without a wheelchair and she is suffering. It is unbearable to see her suffer. We don't really see that giving us another six months with her and watching her suffer and deteriorate in that time is a positive outcome for us.'

I glance over to Claire and double-check that she's still on the same page as me here. She gives me a slight nod and I know she's in agreement.

'We cannot bear the thought of living the rest of our lives knowing there was a chance to save her and we didn't take it. We understand the risks and we understand the challenge, but we really want you to try. We want to be part of this decision and we support you one hundred per cent if you decide to give it a go.'

'Please give her a chance. We know her. She's really

special. We know if you give her a chance, she'll take it,' says Claire.

Jo, Matthew and Fiona all glance at one another for a second and then Jo gives a response. 'We have spoken about this as a team and our feeling is that we would be willing to undertake an assessment laparotomy on Leah. That means we would be willing to get her on the table and open her up to see what can be done.'

Matthew then adds, 'You need to understand that there is a strong chance that we will open Leah up and have a look, and then realise that there is very little we can do and have no option but to sew her back up without attempting anything further.'

'We understand that, Matthew. We are just desperate for you to give her a chance,' I reply.

'I think we need to know that we have your support, and it sounds like we do. Therefore, it sounds like we might have agreed a plan. This will be a complex procedure that will need a fair bit of planning, so it won't happen for a few weeks, but we'll be in touch as soon as possible with a date,' finishes Matthew.

And with that, Claire and I thank the three of them, then thank them again and leave the room.

During the meeting, we heard the words we desperately needed to hear. The surgeons are going to give her a chance! We leave the room clutching onto real, albeit slim, hope once more. The chances of her coming through this operation alive and without any serious damage are frighteningly small, and under normal circumstances that would have been excruciating to hear. However, given that we entered the room expecting the team to tell us there was zero chance, hearing that there is a ten per cent chance feels strangely positive. Ten per cent, after all, is a chance and that is all we could have possibly hoped for.

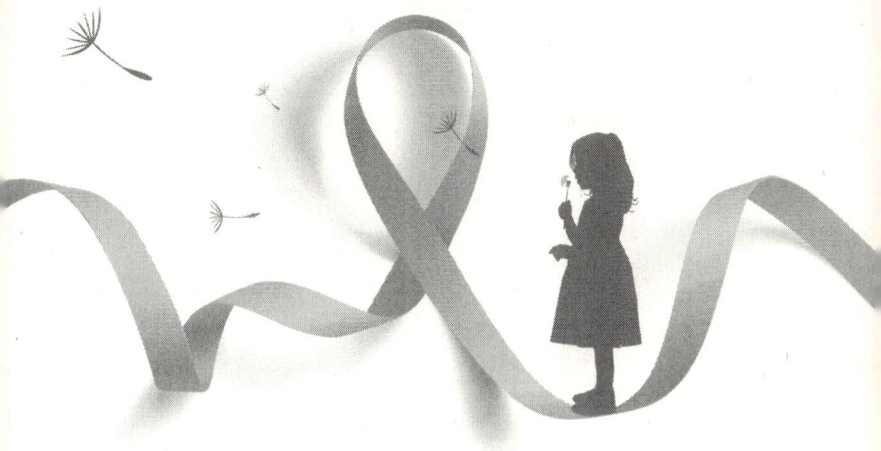

Planning Ahead

Friday 14th June 2019

We receive yet another letter from Alder Hey through the post today. After the last letter, I've really started to question whether it is the right thing to do for my mental health to keep opening and reading them. I suspect this one is the summary of the meeting with the surgeons, so I open it up. It is exactly that letter. I take a deep breath and read it.

Thankfully, there is nothing in the letter that I'm not expecting to read this time, but it does clarify the scale of the risk associated with the operation in quite stark terms.

The chances of Leah making it through this operation are incredibly slim. I'm starting to understand why all the other children's hospitals in the country advised against attempting it. The fact is, though, as black and white as it sounds, if she doesn't survive the operation, then at least we will know that

We would only really know whether surgery were possible by doing an operation (an **assessment laparotomy**), with a view to proceeding with surgery if the situation looked favourable. We estimate that there would be a 80% chance that surgery could not be attempted. In the 20% chance that surgery were possible, the risk of life threatening blood loss would be our major concern. This may be serious enough to cause Leah to die during surgery.

A second very serious complication is damage to the venous drainage of the legs, particularly the left leg, which might result in venous gangrene as the blood flow into the leg eventually comes to a standstill because blood flow out is blocked. Leah would almost certainly die as a result of this happening, although this would not be during surgery itself.

A third major complication would be complete lower limb paralysis due to damage to the spinal cord. Estimates of risk are difficult to give in such uncommon situations, but we feel that the risk of death or serious complication such as paralysis is around 50%.

we gave her every chance. She also won't have to suffer the pain that this disease will give her as it starts to take over her body. We've just lived through that with Marie and to have to support Leah through that is just unimaginable. If she does survive the operation, but she loses the use of her legs and is left in a wheelchair for the rest of her life, then we could also deal with that. We can move house. We can buy a bungalow or perhaps install a lift at the back of our house. What we can't deal with is people giving up and not trying to help her. As terrifying as this situation is, I have absolutely no doubt whatsoever that this is the right thing to do, and I simply cannot allow myself to question that decision.

Barry calls in the afternoon, too. He tells me that he has set us up a meeting with Professor Bannan over in Manchester so that we can speak to her about the plan for Leah's treatment. As soon as the call ends, I open my laptop and open Google to start researching possible treatments to discuss with Prof. Bannan. We've consciously avoided 'Dr Google' so far and I'm glad we have, but now we need to know about anything and everything that might provide a solution for Leah.

Monday 17th June 2019

Claire and I drive across to Manchester Children's Hospital just after lunchtime. We make our way to the oncology outpatient department where we are due to meet Prof. Bannan at 2pm. We arrive a little early and sit in the waiting room. I'm glancing around the room looking at the various colourful displays on the walls that patients have created, when I notice a door with a glass panel to my left. Through the glass panel, I can see a few people in the room and, low and behold, there is Suzie with Jaxon sitting on her knee playing. It warms my heart to see him smiling. *Keep going, little guy*, I think to myself.

Professor Bannan is kind enough to give Claire and I a good half an hour or so to chat through some possible treatment options for Leah and answer a ton of questions we have. She is well aware of the details of Leah's case and is really reassuring with us. I think that is quite a skill in a clinician, especially when it is highly unlikely that they have personal lived experience of what families like ours have to go through. Many of the treatments that we've come across via Google are possible second line chemotherapy drugs that could be suitable for Leah in the future, so this is helpful to know. Professor Bannan reiterates that surgery will undoubtedly give Leah the best chance of survival and she is really pleased to have heard that the Alder Hey surgeons have agreed to give it a go.

She wishes us the very best of luck at the end of the meeting and tells us that she'll check in with Barry to find out how Leah is getting on. Claire and I feel much more positive about things after speaking to her. She has topped up our cup of hope a little and maybe, just maybe, it was now starting to look half full once more.

On the walk back to the car park from the hospital, Claire nudges me and points out two magpies sat together on a fence. We both smile. This helps to top up that cup a little more.

Wednesday 19th June 2019

Today is our second meeting of the week with a brand-new clinician in a completely different hospital. We take Leah across to the Clatterbridge Cancer Centre on the Wirral to meet Dr Thorp. Dr Thorp is also a consultant oncologist, but she specialises in paediatric radiotherapy. We are here to see her to discuss the plan for Leah's radiotherapy treatment, which will be scheduled to commence once she has recovered from the surgery. The fact that the next stages of Leah's treatment is being planned is, in itself, a hugely positive source of hope for Claire and I.

The meeting is actually more intense than I anticipated it might be. As part of the recent Google search, we had explored the potential for Leah to have new proton beam therapy[32]. Unfortunately, Nicky tells us that Leah will not be suitable for that treatment due to the size and location of the tumour in her body. This is a bit of a blow for us.

---

32 Proton Beam Therapy is essentially very similar to traditional radiotherapy treatment, except it is much more precise. It therefore comes without many of the wider side effects that come with radiotherapy.

Nicky then goes on to describe the potential side effects of the radiotherapy treatment. She informs us that there is a high risk of infertility for Leah due to the radiation having to pass through her ovaries. She also informs us that there is a significant risk of renal (kidney) failure due to the fact that her kidneys, and specifically her right kidney, are in close proximity to the tumour and are therefore likely to be within range of the radiation. She goes on to inform us that there is potential for bowel scarring that could possibly cause a bowel obstruction in later life. This could mean that Leah would require a colostomy in adulthood.

Jeez! It is hard to hear all this. I know it is all ifs, buts and maybes, but it is really upsetting to think that she may well be dealing with the negative effects of the treatment for the rest of her life. This treatment, which is the only thing that could save her life, could actually end up cutting her life short or making it really difficult in the future.

We thank Nicky for her time and we both leave the room a little shell-shocked. In truth, the conversation we've just had is irrelevant if she doesn't get through the operation, so I guess we just need to worry about what all this means in due course. It's good to know we have more things to worry about when we've stopped worrying about the things we're currently worried about, though, eh?

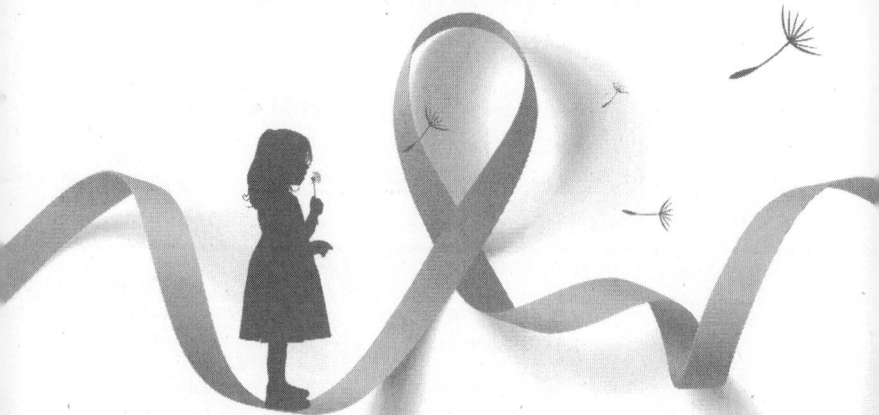

Taking the Piss

Thursday 20th June 2019

Back to the usual routine today as chemo round eight starts. Six more days of fighting with Leah to eat a mouthful of cereal and holding a cardboard sick bowl for her while she vomits it back up ten minutes later. The saddest thing is that Claire and I have become a little numb to the whole thing now. We've normalised it. It is now just how we are required to live life.

As has become the routine, I'm on duty for the first day/night and a combination of Claire, Amy, my sister, Sarah, and I will cover off the remaining days between us.

The nurses come over and hook Leah up to the pumps at around 11:30am, just after she's been checked out by the senior nurse on duty. Leah is surprisingly cheerful today and seems to be in a really chatty mood, which is a nice surprise for being in hospital. We build some Lego together and then start to chat.

Soon, the conversation moves into how she feels about everything that is going on. She talks about her hair falling out. This is not a subject matter that we cover often for obvious reasons, but she is the one dictating the conversation, so I go along with her. She tells me she thought she would be really upset about losing her hair, but she knows it is just a result of the strong medicine that she is taking and it will grow back when she stops taking it. I just sit and listen to her. It is fascinating to hear how someone so young, who is going through something so challenging, has learned to come to terms with it and process it all. I'm in awe of her spirit and courage.

She goes on to tell me that the only time she gets upset about her hair is when strangers look at her funny or call her a boy. She tells me that children are the worst for doing this. I tell her that most children are lucky enough not to understand what she has been through and they also don't understand the impact their words can have.

'I'll never say those things to people, Daddy, because I know how upset it can make them,' she says.

Later that day, as the chemo drugs start to take effect, Leah's chattiness wears off slightly and she also becomes a lot more fatigued. It is so tough to see the difference in her before and after the treatment is started as she retreats into herself. It must be so difficult for her.

Just as we are both settling down for the night, Leah tells me she needs to use the toilet. She is really tired and not in a good mood and she asks me to get a commode for her to use rather than her have to walk across to the bathroom with the pumps on the stand. I pop outside the room to the sluice room, find a clean commode and wheel it back into Leah's room and move it to the side of her bed. It is only then that I realise I don't have any cardboard bowls to place under the commode so that Leah can use it. I pop out of the room to see whether I can find any and I immediately see one of the healthcare assistants on duty tonight. I don't recognise her as one of the regular team, so I presume she is a member of agency staff. I ask her if she can bring us a cardboard bowl to collect urine.

Two minutes later, she returns to the room and hands Leah a cardboard tube to collect urine… for males. She leaves the room. I glance at Leah and she starts to cry. I sit on the bed and give her a cuddle. I think it is a genuine error on behalf of the member of staff and I have no doubt in my mind that she would be horrified to know that she had upset Leah by assuming she was a boy. However, given the conversation that Leah and I had earlier today, it is hard to think that this could have been timed any worse.

Friday 21st June 2019

Last night was a fairly difficult night. Leah was really sick throughout the night and, although she did sleep in between being unwell, she is absolutely shattered this morning, as am I. That was night one of six as well.

At around 2pm, my mobile phone rings. No Caller ID. I answer it; it is Jo Minford. She is calling to ask how Leah is and to inform me that they have agreed a date for

Leah's operation. It will happen on Thursday 1st August. I thank her and end the call. My heart is racing. We have a date. The biggest date of our lives. It is real and I can't quite believe that we've got here, but it seems like we have. I look up to the ceiling.

'Thank you, Marie… and please keep going.'

My sister, Sarah, is up from Birmingham again to stay in with Leah tonight. She comes in to take over from me at 6pm. She has a big bag with her full of goodies for the night. Leah comes to life when Sarah comes in and the pair of them have mischief in their eyes and smiles on their faces as I say goodnight and leave them to it.

I arrive home half an hour later and Claire shows me her phone. It is a WhatsApp photo from Sarah of her and Leah with neon face paint on, sat in a Glastonbury-style yurt made out of bed sheets. I can't help but feel sorry for the nurses on duty tonight dealing with the trouble in room three.

Saturday 22nd June 2019

Claire leaves the house before lunchtime to go and take over from Sarah at the hospital. When she gets there, she sends me a photo of Leah waving to me with the caption, 'Hi, Daddy, I'm feeling good today.' The photo really rocks me because it just doesn't look like her. It doesn't look like my little girl at all. Her eyebrows and eyelashes have now all fallen out and her hair is really thin and wispy.

It's strange that it has taken this photo for me to really notice how much of an impact the last few months have had on her appearance. While I've spent more or less every day by her side since February, to me, she has always looked like my Leah. The child in this photo just looks so poorly and weak. Ironically, in terms of her physical presentation, she seems to be much more mobile and her posture has certainly seemed to improve a little from earlier in the year.

Sunday 23rd June 2019

I'm back on hospital duty tonight. I haven't seen Leah since Friday evening and I've become so naturally protective of her that I struggle when I'm not there with her. I really want to see her, so I can validate that the photo Claire sent me was just a bad shot and she genuinely does not look as ill in reality. I join Claire in the hospital soon after lunchtime. When I get there, Leah gives me a big smile. While she does definitely look pale and poorly, her spirit is not dampened and she still looks beautiful in my eyes.

She seems to be in a mischievous mood and full of beans today and I want to make the most of it. Therefore, after a bit of deliberation, later in the afternoon, we decide to set up a treasure hunt in her room. Leah makes a sequence of eight clues written on different scraps of paper and we hide them around the room. Each clue takes you to the next one. The penultimate clue requires the participant to pull a large plastic 'bogey' out of a plastic head, which makes the head explode and a key fly out of the top[33].

---

33 The plastic head is actually a well-known game called Gooey Louie that Leah has 'adapted'.

The key opens up the 'treasure chest' (aka the toilet roll dispenser) in the bathroom and inside the treasure chest is a small bag of Haribo sweets. Leah is beyond excited about inviting her first victim, sorry, participant to take part. She makes a small notice for me to stick on the door of her room. It says, 'TREASURE HUNT IN HERE'.

Undoubtedly drawn in by the exquisite marketing on the door, a couple of nurses on the ward come in to enquire about what is on offer. They excitedly agree to be willing participants and then eagerly start hunting around the room. Within about five minutes, they have successfully found all the clues and eventually leave with the Haribo bounty from the treasure chest. The bogey-pulling is a particular point of interest for them all and Leah is in absolute hysterics watching them all taking part.

A short time later comes the highlight of the afternoon, when the one and only Big Bad Barry agrees to come in and take part. With a gang of the ward staff watching him from the door, he pulls out the bogey, catches the key, disappears into the bathroom to locate the treasure chest and then emerges thirty seconds later chewing on Haribo to a rapturous round of applause from the audience. I bet he never thought after four years of medical school, ten years as a junior doctor and then probably another twenty or thirty years as a consultant and a professor that his proudest achievement would be winning a small bag of sweets from a toilet roll dispenser! I hope he is proud.

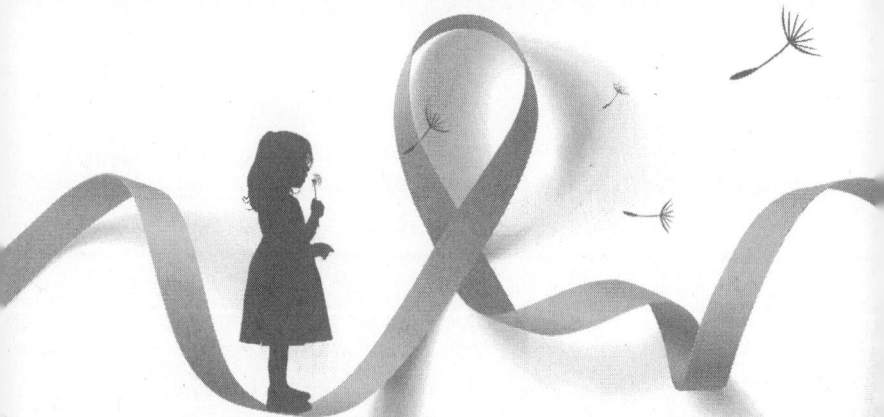

Jelly Bean Roulette

Monday 24th June 2019

Nugget came by to see us today. He was his usual bubbly self and always seems to be able to put a smile on our faces through his natural banter with Leah. The main purpose of his visit is to help us fill some forms that might help us to access some financial grants. A few months ago, he helped us to fill out the ridiculously lengthy and complicated paperwork required to apply for disability allowance for Leah after her initial diagnosis. Now, he is helping us to apply for some other small sources of funding to help a little bit with the household bills etc.

I'm quite lucky that I work for the NHS because I'm covered for full pay for six months while off sick, so we are not desperate for money right now. However, I'm extremely conscious that my pay will drop by half in the coming months and then to nothing from February next year. I also have absolutely no idea how long I will need to stay off work to support Leah, Claire and Phoebe, and I also have no idea how on earth I'm going to pay my mortgage after February if I'm unable to return to work for whatever reason. Therefore, reluctantly, I agree that we probably need to accept any financial help on offer right now, even if it is just to put the money away to help us in the future, if and when we get there.

Nugget helps us fill in grant forms to send to a number of charities who offer financial support to families in our situation. If we are lucky enough to be successful with any of the grant bids, we don't anticipate any of the sums will be hugely significant, but it will all help if and when the time comes when we hit zero pay. I feel really uncomfortable asking these charities for money to help us, but I have to swallow my pride and do what is right for the family.

Also today, yet another charity threw their support our way when a pair of made-to-measure pyjamas and a matching theatre gown were delivered to our home for Leah. The charity that made them is called Pyjama Fairies. They specialise in making bespoke, individual nightwear for children going through difficult times in hospital. It turns out that one of Claire's friends found the charity online and ordered the items on Leah's behalf, so we knew very little about it. We've told Leah that they've arrived and she has already decided that she'd like to wear them when she goes for her operation in August. I'm pleased she is starting to get her head around the fact that she's going back to theatre soon. She is obviously nervous about it, but she acknowledges it is coming up and that is definitely a positive in terms of getting her to go through with it.

Wednesday 26th June 2019

At long, long last, the final day of chemo round eight is here. The six-day stays are just so hard for all of us, especially Leah. She is completely fed up of being in the hospital and fed up of feeling ill and especially fed up of Claire and I. The current bag of drugs is due to finish the infusion at 1:52pm, so once her central lines have been flushed through and they've checked her over one final time, we'll be on our way home, thank God.

1:52pm ticks by and the chemo infusion finishes. Ten minutes later, one of the nurses comes in to disconnect Leah from the pumps and flush her lines through. Thirty minutes later, one of the senior nurses comes in to check her over. She's extremely pale, but her temperature is within the normal levels and her other observations are normal, so they confirm that they are happy to discharge her. We are told that we just need to wait for her medicines to take home with us and then we're good to go. The meds are not quite ready yet, so we'll just have to wait around until they are. Hopefully not too long.

The time is approaching 3pm now, so I pack up our bags and get our few bits of remaining food out of the parent's fridge while we wait.

4pm comes and goes. We are still sat in the room, waiting on the meds.

5pm ticks round. I've asked what the delay is and

apparently they are waiting on one of the doctors to come and formally prescribe the medicines on the system before they can be dispensed. There is no doctor on the ward right now and the surgeon on-call is tied up in theatre. We have no choice but to just sit and wait.

6pm now and we are still here. Leah has fallen asleep. I honestly feel like I want to cry. I'm so tired and pissed off with everything. All I want to do is take her home.

At 6:33pm, over four hours since Leah actually finished the treatment, one of the nurses comes in with the bag of medication and we are finally allowed to go home. It is unbelievably frustrating and I am so angry. All the way home, I am furious about the fact that we've been unnecessarily made to wait over four hours longer than we should have, especially at the end of six gruelling days stuck on the hospital ward for Leah.

The whole experience overshadows the fact that for those six days, Leah has been treated like a princess by the staff and nothing has been too much trouble for them. They've joined in with her games, chatted to her every day and made her feel special. I'm now getting angry with myself for being angry about something so trivial. I need to sleep, clearly.

Friday 28th June 2019

Becky came round to the house yesterday to take Leah's bloods as usual and brought her a present. Leah has previously been telling Becky about her love of all things Harry Potter. Becky had subsequently spotted a small box of 'Bertie Bott's Every Flavour Beans'[34] in a shop and bought them as a nice surprise for her. Leah has since been handing them out to anyone and everyone, and then sitting back to watch their reaction as they realise the flavour. It's like Russian roulette but with jelly beans.

Today, the oncology outreach team are not able to come to our house for Leah's usual GCSF infusion, so we have to take her to the oncology day care ward to have it done there. The opportunity to cause some mischief with the box of Bertie Bott's beans is not lost on Leah, of course.

We make our way to the hospital and as soon as we walk onto the ward, Leah starts scanning for victims… no, volunteers to sample the jelly beans. Most of the ward clerks and nurses suspect they are not normal jelly beans and promptly refuse. One of the more gregarious nurses, and another of Leah's favourites, Karen, agrees to try one. Leah watches her reaction closely. She whispers to me that she spotted the colour of the bean as Karen picked it. According to her, it is either watermelon or cinnamon. Karen confirms it tastes like watermelon and she seems happy with that. Leah looks disappointed.

Shortly after that, Leah is hooked up to the syringe driver to commence the GCSF. While she is sat there waiting for the syringe driver to complete its duties, who should walk past and say hello? Nugget.

Bingo! He is an absolute prime candidate for a jelly bean. I almost feel sorry for him. I suspect there is no way

---

34 'Every Flavour' being the operative words. The box contains beans flavoured with everything from banana to earwax and marshmallow to vomit.

he's avoiding this. I think he senses there is no escape and he agrees to give one a go. He picks a white-ish coloured bean and pops it in his mouth. I look at Leah and she is staring at him, smirking.

What happens next can only be described as carnage. His face immediately suggests that he has chosen a less favourable flavour. His eyes shoot around the ward area as he realises that he has nowhere to spit it out. He starts running round with his face screwed up, making baulking noises. It is so funny. Leah is rolling around laughing, as are a number of the staff around the ward.

Eventually, someone takes pity on him and offers him a tissue to deposit the bean in.

'What was that you gave me, Miss Leah?' asks Nugget.

'Rotten egg!' screams Leah, still in hysterics.

Ten minutes later, Big Bad Barry saunters past. This is almost too good to be true. I'm more excited about this than Leah. She shouts him over and offers him a jelly bean. He reaches into the tub and picks out a purple one. We all stare at him, waiting for the reaction. In my head, I'm screaming, 'Vomit flavour, *please* be vomit flavour.'

'Mmm, that tastes like cherry,' he says. 'Thank you.' And off he trots.

I'm absolutely gutted.

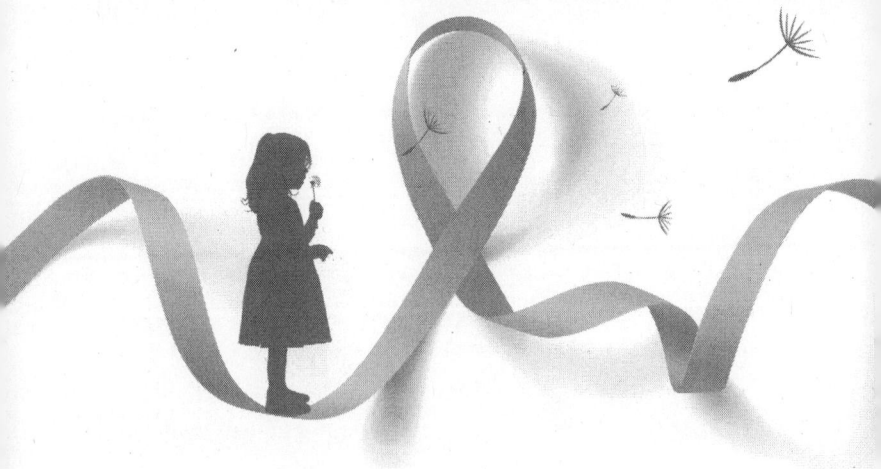

The Power of Kindness

I mentioned earlier in the book about how important hope became for me and for those around me. I also mentioned that we'd all found hope in different ways. Through faith, luck, unerring positivity and even simply through the number of magpies sat on a fence at any one time! However, perhaps the biggest source of hope for me, personally, has come from the words and actions of those around me. I draw strength and inspiration (largely subconsciously, in truth) from the people I encounter on a daily basis. Without even realising it sometimes, the people around me have become my stars in the dark.

Over the last few months in particular, I have found the power of kindness and human compassion to be one of the greatest sources of positivity and hope that I could ever need. One such example stands out above all others, too.

It is early July and Claire has already climbed out of bed to attend morning mass at church. She has been going to church much more often since her mum passed away. Despite all her worries and her questions, she is clearly still finding inner strength from her faith in some way.

While she is out, the doorbell rings at home. I am in the kitchen, drying the dishes, so I throw the tea towel over my shoulder and go to answer the door. When I open it, one of my best friend's mother-in-law is standing there.

'Hello, Nora,' I say in surprise.

I don't ever recall Nora coming to our house before. I didn't know she knew where we lived.

'Would you like to come in? Claire isn't back from church yet, but you're welcome to come in if you would like a cup of tea.'

'Oh… no thank you, Ste. I'm not stopping. Colin [her husband] is in the car, waiting,' she replies. 'We've just popped round to give you this.' She places a white envelope in my hand. 'I know you will probably not want to accept it, but we really want you to take it and do with it whatever you need it for.'

I glance down at the envelope she placed in my hand. It has the name of a bank on it. I'm guessing it therefore contains money that she's giving to us.

'I… I don't know what to say, Nora,' I stutter.

'Please just say that you will accept it and know that we are thinking of you all,' she says assertively.

I look her in the eye and I start to well up. The sheer kindness and generosity of people is just incredible. I feel overwhelmed by it at that moment in time. Nora notices my eyes glaze over and starts to get emotional, too. She turns away from me and makes her way down the drive.

'Good luck with everything and know we are here for you,' she shouts over her shoulder.

'Thank you. Thank you so much,' I say and she jumps in the car at the end of the drive as I close the front door.

I walk back into the kitchen and place the envelope on the worktop. I'm not sure what to do with it. Eventually, around ten minutes later, I decide to open the envelope. It contains a thousand pounds. I cry again. I am totally stunned. A thousand pounds is certainly not an insignificant amount of money to most people who live near us, and I don't think for a second that this does not apply to Nora and Colin. It is quite simply the most incredibly kind gesture I've ever witnessed.

Claire comes home twenty minutes later and I tell her about Nora and Colin coming round. I hand her the envelope and she looks inside. She cries, too.

Right there is an amazing example of seeing those stars in the dark sky yet again. People who go out of their way to do something, anything, to help. People who don't need to do it and I would not think any less of, if they had chosen not to do this. People who just want you to know that they are supporting you and they care.

Sending a small message of support, donating your hair to a charity, running a marathon to raise money or even painting someone's pet dog on a pair of converse shoes[35]. All of these acts of kindness make a huge difference when you're going through tough times. I would argue they can sometimes be the reason that people make it through.

---

35 Note: only if you're a good artist – I tried drawing our pet pug once and it looked more like the poo emoji.

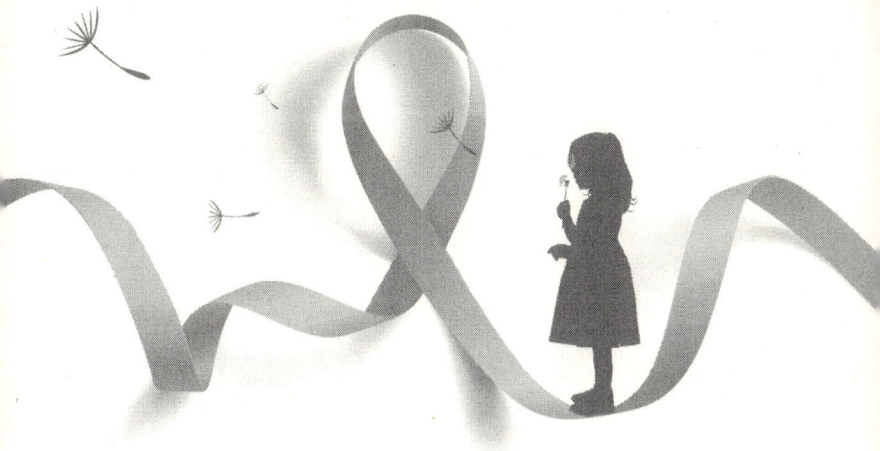

Cops and Robbers

Thursday 4th July 2019

It is my turn to stay with Leah in her room. I switch on her feed pump and give her medicine just before bed, as is the usual routine now. I set the usual alarms to wake me up at regular intervals throughout the night to give her the other meds and check her temperature etc.

At 1:50am, her feed pump on the table next to her bed beeps to tell me it has finished and the bottle is empty. I roll out of bed half asleep and disconnect the tubing from Leah's PEG and flush it with a small amount of water. Just before I jump back into bed, I do the usual temperature check. The display on the digital thermometer glows amber and flashes up 38.1°C. Oh, please no.

I peel back her bed sheets slightly and let her cool down a little, then two minutes later, I check again. Still 38.1°C.

The clock is close to ticking past 2am and every single bone in my body desperately wants this thermometer to read a normal level so I can go back to sleep. The thermometer has become a symbol of dread for me and it is defiantly sticking resolutely to the 38.1°C figure. I know I have no choice but to take her into the hospital. I go and wake Claire up to let her know. I then get myself dressed, gather up the overnight bags, scoop Leah half asleep out of bed and carry her downstairs to the car.

We join the M62 and head towards Liverpool. It is 2:20am. Leah is dozing in the passenger seat. I am barely awake and bleary-eyed. I am so sick of having to do all this. I call Ward 3B and alert them that we are on the way to A&E. This is the standard protocol in this situation. It is almost exactly a week since she finished her latest round of chemo, which means her bloods are likely to be at risky levels. I start to fantasise that the A&E staff will tell me that our thermometer is broken and her temperature is actually fine so we can turn round and go straight home.

As we approach the junction where we usually leave the motorway, there is a line of red lights on the road ahead and blue flashing lights at the front of them. I become much more alert immediately. I have no idea what this is, but it doesn't feel great. Leah wakes up next to me and is inquisitive, too. As I draw closer, it becomes clear that the police have stopped the traffic on the motorway. There must be some kind of incident on the slip road and roundabout that we were looking to come off at.

I pull up at the back of the small queue of traffic. I start to get nervous. I know Leah's temperature is up and

I know that means we have to get her into A&E as quickly as possible. I also know her blood count will probably be low and those two things can be a dangerous combination. I have no idea how long they are intending to hold the traffic. After sitting anxiously in the queue of traffic for about five minutes, I make the decision to drive down the hard shoulder and bypass the queue of cars, ignoring the angry faces of the other drivers as I do. When I reach the front, I swerve across to line up my car with the police car sat holding up the other cars.

The police officer in the driver's seat winds down the passenger window as I wind down my window. He has a face like absolute thunder and is looking at me as if he about to scream in my face. I point out to him that I urgently need to get off the motorway to get my daughter to hospital.

'The road is closed off for now. You will have to wait,' he replies.

'I understand that,' I say, 'but my daughter has cancer and is unwell and it is really urgent that I get her to Alder Hey as quickly as possible.'

He looks me in the eye as if testing out whether I'm being genuine. I mean, for Christ's sake, nobody is going to make up a story like that just to jump a traffic queue, surely?! The officer arches his neck forward and looks past me to see Leah in the passenger seat in her dressing gown looking fairly unwell. If he still thinks I've made this all up now, this guy really does see the worst in people.

He radios ahead to a colleague on the slip road in the distance. I can hear him pushing his colleague, who clearly is not interested in letting anyone through. In the end, they agree to allow us through. I thank him and drive slowly onwards and up the slip road. At the top, there are pieces of car scattered all over the road. I can see a good number of police officers in hi-vis yellow jackets searching with torches in the trees at the side of the roundabout for something. I drive slowly through the debris, dodging fragments of headlights and wing mirrors on the road. Leah is absolutely wide awake now. In fact, she is hanging out of the window, excitedly looking for a criminal who she is adamant must be hiding in the trees. I'm certain the police officers who saw us drive past are now convinced we've made up our whole story after seeing Leah waving at them.

We made it to Alder Hey ten minutes later. Our thermometer is sadly not broken. Leah's temperature is indeed over 38°C. Her bloods are indeed at dangerous levels. We make it up to Ward 3B just after 4am and we're staying in for the next two days. Leah never did find the criminal.

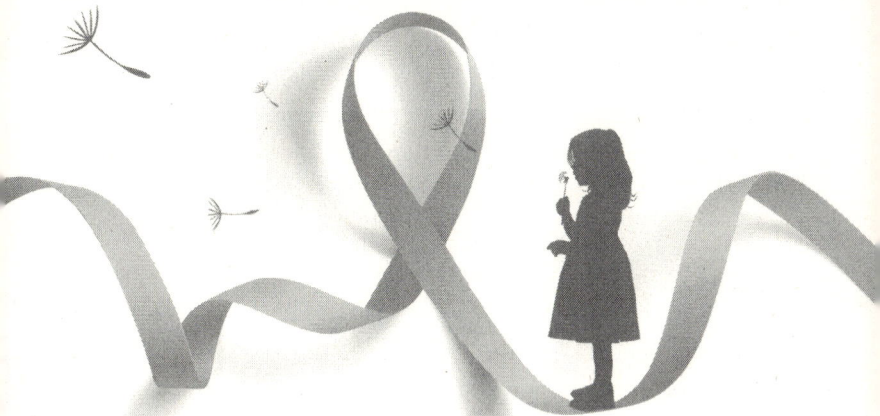

Pre-flight Checks (and Chinese Food)

Sunday 7th July 2019

I'm in Leah's room, sorting out the drawers where we keep all the syringes, plasters and other medical paraphernalia for her care. I have just finished checking the dates on the various bottles of medicine on top of the chest of drawers when I turn round too quickly and knock the bloody Bella statue onto the floor *again*! I roll my eyes and then bend down to pick up the pieces from the floor. She is pretty badly damaged this time and I'm not sure it is fixable. I place the pieces in the bin in the corner of the room. Leah will be fuming with me when she finds out.

I go downstairs and flick the kettle on. As I stand waiting for it to boil, I think about the little Bella statue. Bella has been broken so many times from so many different sources. I shake my head and chuckle to myself about the number of times I've now attempted to fix it. I then start to think about Leah. I then start to think about Leah and Bella, and I wonder whether Bella has possibly become a metaphor for Leah's own fight. After all, we've had to continually pick her up and try our best to fix her. I start to get emotional thinking about it, to the point that I go straight back upstairs and fish the various pieces back out of the bin. I take the pieces downstairs, place them on the kitchen table and then fetch the superglue.

Once I've finished gluing Bella back together once more, I stand her on the table in front of me. There are a few tiny pieces missing and some of the breaks are visible. Just like Leah, she has a few scars and signs of wear and tear, but she is standing back up with a smile on her face and holding her wand proudly. We've all come too far to give up now and that includes Bella.

Thursday 11th July 2019

Today, we are back in the hospital for the start of Leah's ninth round of chemotherapy. Her big operation is now just three weeks away. Barry has reduced the dose for this round to give her the best possible chance of recovering in time.

Friday 12th July 2019

Leah has had an awful lot of weird and wonderful tests across the course of the day today. She's been down to the cardiology department for an echo test on her heart. She has also had some kind of kidney function test, which required her to have blood samples taken every hour for a few hours. It is all in preparation for the upcoming surgery. She is like an astronaut about to be launched into space and they are doing the pre-flight checks.

The way she is able to take all this in her stride is testament to her strength and resilience – two traits that she has in abundance and she will need to draw upon these over the next few weeks. We all will.

Sunday 14th July 2019

What is hopefully and possibly Leah's final ever chemotherapy session finished today. The last three days have passed by without any major issues and Leah has coped better with this round of treatment than most of the others. All of our focus is now on the 1st August. We have to wrap her in cotton wool between now and then, so that she is in the best possible condition for that operation and to give her the best possible chance to get through.

Claire has already stepped up the prayers and I'm really starting to feel the magnitude of the situation. I'm so nervous and feel constantly anxious at the moment, but I know in my heart we cannot do any more now. We know she has it in her to overcome this, but we just need luck to be on her side, too.

Tuesday 16th July 2019

We are required to take Leah in for an MRI scan today. My understanding of the purpose of this scan is so that the surgeons have the most up-to-date images of what they are taking on. She doesn't flinch when she is pulled out of the machine to have the dye injected for the final part of the scan today. Instead, she just turns her head away when the needle goes into her arm. She has grown so much in so many ways over the last six months, it is just incredible. She's shown maturity and strength that is way, way beyond her years.

When we get home from the hospital, there are a couple of letters on the doormat for us. One from the Family Fund charity and the other from Fletcher's Fund. Both contain cheques for us to help us pay for things for Leah that we might be struggling with under the circumstances. These are some of the charities that Nugget approached for us. It is very humbling to open these envelopes and know that people have fundraised and donated to these charities to allow them to help families like mine.

I look up Fletcher's Fund on the internet as I'm conscious I don't know an awful lot about them. It turns out they are a small charity based up in Carlisle, which was set up by a family after they lost their young son, Fletcher, to cancer a few years ago. Incredible, inspirational people who have been through the unimaginable and are determined to make a difference to others in that situation. If only the world had more people like them, I suspect we would have already found a cure for this fucking awful disease by now.

Wednesday 17th July 2019

It is Phoebe's birthday. A day she has been so excited for since Boxing Day last year. It is also a day when we get the chance to put her in the spotlight for once. No, actually, it is a day when we *need* to put her in the spotlight. We asked her a few weeks ago what she wanted to do for her birthday and she said she wanted to take a group of her friends to play laser tag – so that's exactly what we're doing.

The problem this causes is that Leah wants to join in, too, and we're not sure that this is a good idea. Her physical condition has improved dramatically over the last couple of months considering she couldn't sit upright in a chair back in March/April. She is probably okay to play a game with Phoebe and her friends, but she still has a central line and a PEG tube in her body. The thought of her running round in the dark and bumping into one of Phoebe's friends and something happening is a real concern. However, Claire and I both know it will take a minor miracle to stop her!

The solution? Peter has already sorted it for her. He has hand-made a padded vest for her to wear to cover over her front. It fits her perfectly. Nothing is now stopping her from going into the arena and shooting Phoebe and her friends. Knowing Leah, though, she'll mainly be shooting Phoebe.

Not only does she want to join in with one of the games of laser tag, but she ends up playing all three games. She is completely soaked with sweat when she comes out and she is exhausted, but she absolutely loves it. It is a brilliant evening. Phoebe has a great time; her friends all seem to love it; and Leah, for one evening, is as far away from the hospital as she's been in many, many months.

Friday 26th July 2019

Claire and I have to go into the hospital today to see Barry about the results of Leah's latest MRI scan. Of course, the traffic lights outside the hospital are on red when we roll up. It's become a bit of a running joke between Claire and I now.

I'm not sure whether or not the results of this scan matter too much in terms of the decision to operate, but I certainly don't feel as anxious about hearing them today for some reason. I think Claire feels the same as she's agreed to come with me, and she doesn't seem to be on edge. Certainly not as much as she has been before when we've gone to receive news from Barry.

Barry tells us that the scan results have suggested a further small reduction in the size of the tumour. This is great to hear and I guess any remaining doubt about whether the surgeons might change their minds has surely now been extinguished. It is a strange feeling walking out of the clinic room after the meeting with Barry. It felt almost like a non-event in some ways. We are so completely focused on the 1st August now that the days are feeling blurred and we just need to get to that point.

In the evening, I go into Leah's room to tuck her into bed. We have a little chat about the day as usual and I kiss her on the head and give her a big hug.

'I feel safe in your arms, Daddy,' she says to me.

I pause for a second before replying, 'I'm always here, sweetheart. I will always protect you.'

I'm holding her so close she can't see the tears rolling down my cheeks.

Saturday 27th July 2019

It's Saturday morning and I've come down to make breakfast for everyone. Claire is standing next to me while I make the cups of tea and she pulls up the blinds on the kitchen window. The sunlight bursts in. It is a beautiful morning.

'What's that on the garden, Ste?' asks Claire in a puzzled tone.

I lean forward and squint my eyes to focus on the small dark object lying on the grass.

'I'm not sure. It wasn't there yesterday,' I reply.

'I think it looks… like a bird of some kind,' Claire responds.

I glance out of the window again and I think she might be right. Lying in a highly unnatural state on the garden is definitely what looks to be some sort of bird. I unlock the back door and go out to investigate. Sure enough, on the grass next to the raised wooden decked area is a dead bird and… it's only a bloody magpie!

Under normal circumstances, I would probably find this quite upsetting. However, we are in far from normal circumstances at the moment and this is the one bird that has almost symbolised everything about Leah's journey. To see one lying dead on our back garden in the week before the biggest day of our lives is just so strange. Is it a sign or a symbol of our sorrow finally being laid to rest? Did Marie put this here? Do I still just overthink everything at the moment? 'Who knows' is the answer to the first two questions. Yes is most certainly the answer to the third.

Wednesday 31st July 2019

It is the day before Leah's operation. Claire and I have decided that there is absolutely nothing that any of us can do now to affect the outcome tomorrow aside from stay positive and keep hoping and praying that Leah is safe. We've invited both of our close families out for dinner tonight at Leah's favourite local Chinese restaurant. It was not an easy decision to make. In many ways, it might be better to just stay at home and focus on tomorrow. However, as heartbreaking and blunt as this might sound, we're conscious that this may be the last time our families get to see her if things don't go well tomorrow. We want to give everyone the chance to see her smile, to hug her and to tell her that they love her at least one more time.

We arrive at the restaurant later that evening and there is a really strange atmosphere. Every other table has people sitting around, chatting and laughing, but it is like I can't see them. I can't see anything clearly beyond the tables that we are sat on. I just sit watching Leah and watching mine and Claire's families interact with her. I'm thinking constantly about whether this is truly the last time we will all be together. It feels surreal. I hardly eat a thing and I think Claire eats even less.

After the meal, one of the waiting staff brings out a plate full of fortune cookies. Leah and Phoebe take the first two and then, one by one, everyone else around the table takes one, too, leaving the final two on the plate for Claire and I. Claire opens hers before me and immediately shoots me a look of surprise. She passes me the small piece of paper that was folded up inside the cookie and I read it. *Hope is like food; you will starve without it.*

She smiles at me. She has a little tear in her eye.

'It's as if someone gave me that personally,' she says. I know by 'someone', she means her mum.

'Leah, can I see your fortune cookie, please?' I ask and she comes over to me and shows me her note, too.

I am completely stunned by what I read. *Remember that adversity is not a dead end but a detour to a better outcome.*

I know there are probably twenty people who will have read the exact same message from a fortune cookie this week, but the fact that Claire and Leah had been given those exact messages was incredible. I'm the one with a tear in my eye now as I show Claire the message in Leah's cookie.

The time comes for us to leave the restaurant and go back home. One by one, our family members say goodbye and each give Leah the biggest hug ever.

'Be brave tomorrow, Leah,' they say, 'and we'll see you as soon as you are allowed visitors.'

Everyone is trying to be positive and upbeat in front of her, but I can see they are all terrified by the realisation that they could have just spoken to her and hugged her for the last time.

Phoebe jumps into my mum and dad's car. She is staying at their house tonight as we have to be in the hospital early. I give her a huge hug and kiss, and tell her to be good for Nan and Granddad and I'll see her tomorrow. She gives Leah a cuddle, too, and tells her to be brave. I don't think she has any real idea about how significant this moment is, but I'm also kind of glad that she doesn't.

Just before we get into the car outside, my mum comes over to me and gives me the biggest hug she has ever given me. She is visibly upset. This starts me off again.

'Good luck tomorrow, love. We'll all be thinking of you. I love you all so much.'

'We love you, too, Mum,' I reply. I can barely get the words out.

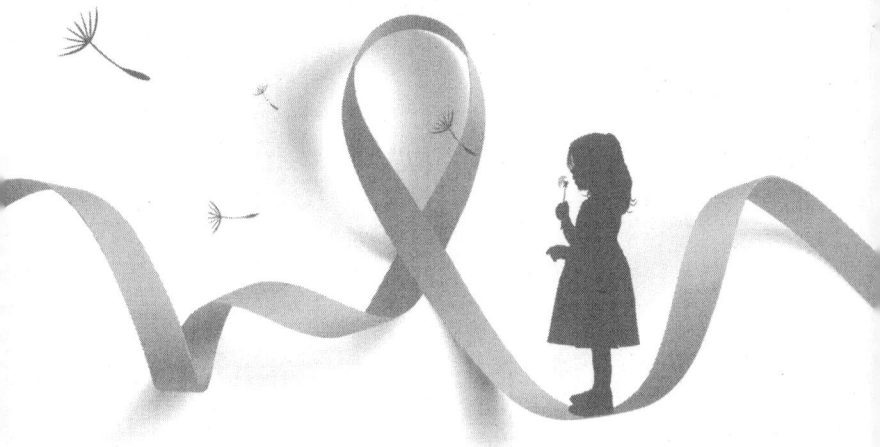

It's Now or Never

Thursday 1st August 2019 – 6:30am

The alarm at the side of the bed bleeps loudly to signify the time is 6:30am. It needn't have wasted its time. I've been wide awake for the last hour. I have a million and one things racing through my brain. I don't think it is any over-exaggeration to say that today is the biggest day of our lives.

I'm immensely proud of everyone involved that we've made it here to this point. The fact that we still have hope that Leah might somehow find a way through all this is alone a huge accomplishment. However, it will count for nothing if she doesn't survive the operation. For that fact alone, I'm completely terrified. There is a real chance, in fact, if the odds are to be believed, that today will be the last day we get to spend with Leah, as a family of four.

I cannot bear to think of what life might look like tomorrow. I just have to keep stopping myself from wandering too far down certain paths again. Get her into that theatre and we give her every chance possible – that is all we can do. The rest is in the hands of others, maybe including Marie.

Getting Leah out of bed is the first battle of the day. Not only is she shattered and hates getting up early, but she also knows what today has in store for her[36]. After a tag team effort between Claire and I, we eventually manage to persuade her to play ball. I pack the car up with Leah's bag and our overnight bags, as we have no idea what the plan will be for tonight. We do know that Leah will be kept on intensive care post-operatively tonight if they decide to attempt the surgery. Regardless of what happens today, Claire and I will need be with each other tonight as we will definitely need to support each other through any possible outcome. We set off for Alder Hey just after 7am.

Thursday 1st August 2019 – 7:30am

The car is quiet as we drive to the hospital. I glance across to Claire in the passenger seat and squeeze her knee every so often, just to say I'm here and we've got this. Each time, she touches my hand and smiles at me faintly.

As we approach the hospital entrance, we enter the

---

36 She knows she is going to theatre, but Claire and I have been careful to avoid a conversation about how big this operation is and what it might all mean. If she really knew, there would be zero chance of getting her into that theatre. She just knows that today they are going to try and remove her 'lump'.

usual filter lane to take us across the opposite side of the road and into the hospital grounds. For quite possibly the first time ever, the traffic light is green and we drive straight through. Even Leah notices from the back seat.

'Daddy, the light is green today! Hooray!' A coincidence? A positive omen? Another sign from Marie to tell us everything is going to be okay? I don't know, but I puff out my chest and take a small burst of positive energy and hope from the thought.

'Come on. She's going to be okay,' I say to myself.

After parking the car, we grab Leah's bag and make our way over to the theatre reception. We give in our details and then head into the waiting area. Leah's height and weight are taken by one of the theatre team and the usual set of observations are completed. After that, we are shown into a small side room where we sit and wait.

About twenty minutes later, the anaesthetist, Dr Ravi, comes in to speak to us. She checks Leah is okay and goes through the paperwork and consent forms with Claire and I. We had spoken to her and Ms Minford last week when they had talked us through the consent forms and given us the opportunity to ask any final questions. There is nothing more we need to know or ask now. We can only wait for Leah to be called in.

Thursday 1st August 2019 – 10am

There is a knock on the door. We look up and two members of the theatre staff enter the room.

'Okay, Leah, we're ready for you,' they say.

My heart rate rises immediately. This is it. This is the moment that we've been desperate to get to for the last six months. This is the moment that determines the path of our lives forever. I'm completely overwhelmed by the enormity of this moment. I know I have to contain and control my emotions so as not to panic Leah any more than she is panicking already. Claire grabs hold of Leah's hand tightly. They fix their gaze on each other. I'm not sure who is reassuring who, but there are no words spoken between them. No words are needed.

Leah turns to me and asks me to carry her into the anaesthetic room. I agree without hesitation. I scoop her up and hold her close to me, squeezing her so tightly so she feels safe. We make our way down the corridor with Claire alongside us, stroking Leah's hair and reassuring her.

'Everything is going to be okay, baby,' she says to Leah. 'Daddy and I will be there to see you as soon as you wake up.'

We enter the anaesthetic room. There is electricity in the air. I can feel it. I can feel this is a big deal. I can feel that this is a big moment for lots of people, not just Leah, Claire and me. There are five people in the anaesthetic room with us. The only one I recognise is Dr Ravi. I assume the others are members of the theatre team. They welcome us in and are as calming and reassuring as possible, but my heart is beating out of my chest.

Leah is wearing her special theatre gown. She looks so frightened and so fragile, yet I know she has an inner strength that can move mountains. She has demonstrated that every time she's been asked to.

I need you to show that strength again, baby girl, I'm thinking. *I also need you to give me some of it.*

She makes it clear to the team in the room that she doesn't want to lie on the bed so they agree that she can sit on Claire's knee while they administer the anaesthetic. I'm hoping that she copes with this situation better than she has in the past. I don't want her to do anything that might jeopardise the procedure at this late stage. She seems much calmer than last time. It is almost like she knows just how important this is and she's accepting it.

'Night, night, Mummy. I love you and I'll see you soon,' she says. Claire hugs her tightly and tells her she loves her. 'I love you, Daddy. I'll see you soon, too,' she then says to me.

'I love you so much, sweetheart,' I just about manage to respond in a whimper.

Dr Ravi pushes the plunger down on the syringe into the back of Leah's hand. Her eyes roll back in her head and the team step in around us to take her now floppy body off Claire's knee. They lie her gently on the trolley, ready to be wheeled into the theatre through the doors behind us.

'Well done, Mum and Dad,' one of the theatre staff says to us. 'Give her a kiss and we'll look after her now.'

I glance around the room. The whole experience seems to be emotional for others, too, as one or two of the theatre team are wiping away tears from their eyes.

Claire kisses Leah on the forehead and strokes her face. She is sobbing her heart out. I then kiss Leah on the cheek and just stare at her beautiful face for a second. I don't want to leave her. I don't want to walk out of that room. I honestly don't know whether I will ever see her alive again. This awful, evil disease has served up some pretty horrendous moments for us these last few months, but having to walk out of this room and leave her behind in these circumstances tops the lot. My heart hurts so much.

Thursday 1st August 2019 – 10:20am

We nervously and reluctantly leave the anaesthetic room. Outside the room, there are a large number of people buzzing around. One of them is Pip, the play specialist from Ward 3B. Pip spent some time sat with us this morning, helping to ensure Leah was calm and suitably distracted before she was called to theatre. She comes straight up to us as we leave the room and throws her arms around us.

'Well done,' she stutteringly says. She has tears in her eyes, too.

Jo Minford then steps forward from the group. 'Don't worry, we'll look after her for you,' she says and she touches Claire's arm reassuringly.

'I know you will,' says Claire through the tears.

'We believe in you. Thank you so much,' I add through my own tears.

Jo then asks us whether we are happy to consent to Leah's procedure being videoed and broadcast into a neighbouring theatre. She explains that this is because there is a lot of interest in the case as it is so complex and unique. The surgical team do not want to be distracted by people coming in and out of the theatre during the day, so they think this is the best option. Of course we agree. If Jo Minford says that gambling our life savings on Mexico winning the *Eurovision Song Contest* is the best option right now, I would do it in a heartbeat.

Jo thanks us and says she will get some sort of contact out to us about the progress of the operation as soon as she can. She tells us that it will be a long procedure and therefore not to necessarily expect to hear anything until maybe lunchtime. With a soft smile, she then turns and disappears back into the anaesthetic room. Claire and I are led back down the corridor to the room where we left Leah's belongings.

When we get there, we just stand in the middle of the room, holding one another. All of the emotion that we've been storing up all morning then pours out of us both.

Thursday 1st August 2019 – 10:45am

After eventually composing ourselves, we gather up our things and decide to go and grab a coffee. We've been told that the theatre has been booked out for a full three-session day and the surgeons have prepped the theatre team that the procedure could take a long time.

The first part of the surgical plan is for Harriet Corbett (a consultant paediatric urologist and another amazing human being) to remove and replace Leah's urethral stents. They have been in situ approaching six months now and need to be replaced. Once Harriet has done her thing, the surgical team will pause and review the plan, and the situation in front of them. If appropriate, they will then open Leah's abdomen and assess the tumour inside. Only then can they really make a decision around whether or not they have any chance of removing it and handing her a chance of survival. Regardless of the decision, Harriet will come out of the theatre and call Claire or myself to update us on the next steps. That moment already feels like it could be life-changing.

Claire and I are sat in Costa Coffee in the main atrium in the hospital. We're a little shell-shocked, in truth. Every minute of this morning so far has been intense and filled with emotion. We are now trying to catch our breaths. The sheer scale of the moment starts to become clear to me as we sit here hugging a latte each. The surgical team involved today consists of Jo, Matthew and Fiona, the three surgeons we met back in June, alongside two anaesthetists and an extensive team of theatre practitioners. Additionally, Ms Corbett is involved, and the group has been joined by Professor John Brennan, a vascular specialist from the Royal Liverpool Hospital. He has agreed to help provide expert advice and guidance around Leah's vascular system. Given the complex and dangerous location of the tumour, this expertise could prove to be vital in terms of ensuring adequate blood flow to and from her lower limbs.

I have worked in hospitals for most of my career and one thing I have learned during that time is that getting more than one surgeon for an operation is a rare occurrence. Therefore, getting four from Alder Hey, as well as a professor of vascular surgery from another local hospital is quite extraordinary. The surgical team use the 3D model that they showed us during the meeting in June to prepare their possible approach to the procedure and to explain to the theatre team what they should expect and the desired outcome. They have set up cameras so that they can allow others to observe and learn from such a significant procedure. It all just demonstrates the lengths these people are prepared to go to in order to give our little girl a fighting chance. I'm sick to my stomach about the sheer magnitude of the events, but also feeling very humbled.

Thursday 1st August 2019 – 11:30am

Trying to distract my mind from something so significant and so important is proving extremely difficult to do. Claire snaps at me for constantly glancing down at my phone. Every time I do it, she thinks it might be someone ringing with some news. She is on edge, too.

We finish our coffees and Claire asks whether I will come with her to the hospital chapel. She wants to pray and ask for help in her way. I always feel slightly fraudulent entering a place of worship when I've never really committed to being a believer, but I agree nonetheless. The chapel at Alder Hey is in a beautiful, slightly quirky wooden treehouse-type structure on the far side of the main atrium of the hospital. I tentatively enter and Claire follows behind. Inside, there is a small altar/lectern facing a small number of rows of wooden seats. To my left, there is a small ornamental metal tree. To my right, there is a barefoot Muslim gentleman, praying on a prayer mat. It is very quiet inside with just the low hum of the Muslim gentleman's words.

Claire takes a seat on one of the rows of seats to the left and I sit down next to her. She immediately closes her eyes, bows her head and begins to pray. I sit in silence next to her, looking out of the window into the bustling atrium of the hospital below. I cannot hear any noise coming from that space through the window, yet there are many people moving around and talking down there. The chapel is a beautiful sanctuary of calm in an otherwise hectic building. It is perfectly peaceful and the light entering the window illuminates it evangelically. Hats off to the designers, who have certainly nailed the brief.

My thoughts switch back to religion and I start to question why I don't feel the need to pray myself. I suppose if my words do fall on deaf ears, then I haven't really lost anything other than my time. Time is one thing I have a lot of today. On the other hand, if my words are heard and listened to, maybe, just maybe, they might make a positive difference. I decide I have nothing to lose, so I bow my head, too, and I ask God to help us and to take care of Leah.

My prayer is complete in five minutes. I raise my head. Claire is still hard at it. I don't want to distract her, so I sneak quietly over to the metal tree in the corner of the room to see what it is. As I get closer, I realise there are numerous pieces of multicoloured paper attached to the branches. On closer examination, they are all handwritten notes. I read a yellow one on the end of the branch closest to me.

Please take care of my grandson on ward 4A. He is very sick and I am scared and I pray that you will keep him safe.

The rest of the notes on the branches follow a similar theme. It feels strangely powerful to be standing here reading them. Stood on the very spot where each of these people have stood and identified another small source of hope. I decide to add a note of my own. I pick up a pen and a small piece of yellow paper. I ask for help in getting Leah through her operation and in giving Claire and I the strength to keep going, no matter what happens today. I hang the note on one of the branches. I feel better for doing it.

Ten minutes later and Claire is finished, so we make our way back out of the chapel. It is rapidly approaching lunchtime, but neither of us is able to stomach any food. I decide to go and purchase a small bottle of water and we agree it might be helpful for us to get out of the hospital for a while to get some fresh air. Alder Hey is built right next to a small park, so we head outside and across there. The park has a pathway running round the outer perimeter, so we follow that, wherever it ends up taking us.

We get about halfway round and Claire nudges me and points out that two magpies have just landed on the grass to our right. I smile. I feel so anxious today that I dread to think what state I would be in had it only been one single bird. We proceed to walk four laps of the park, talking and sharing our thoughts, fears and hopes. All the way round, I constantly check my phone to make sure I have a signal in case we receive a call.

I was hoping we would have heard something by now.

Thursday 1st August 2019 – 1:36pm

We make our way out of the park and decide to sit down on a bench outside the front entrance of the hospital. It's a great place to people-watch. We sit and watch mums, dads and grandparents of all shapes, sizes, races and religions, walking into and out of the hospital. They are pushing prams, holding hands with their kids and some have a familiar look of frustration on their faces as their children follow at least ten steps behind them, walking at a snail's pace. They all have their own stories and their own reasons for being here. I wonder whether any of these people are the others who have added notes to the tree in the chapel. I wonder whether any of them are waiting on news of their child in theatre. I wonder whether any of them have faced losing their child and, if so, how they coped with those thoughts and emotions.

My wandering mind is interrupted by my phone going off in my pocket. I immediately grab it and look at the screen – No Caller ID.

'Hello,' I say, perhaps a little too eagerly.

'Hello, Stephen. It's Harriet Corbett.'

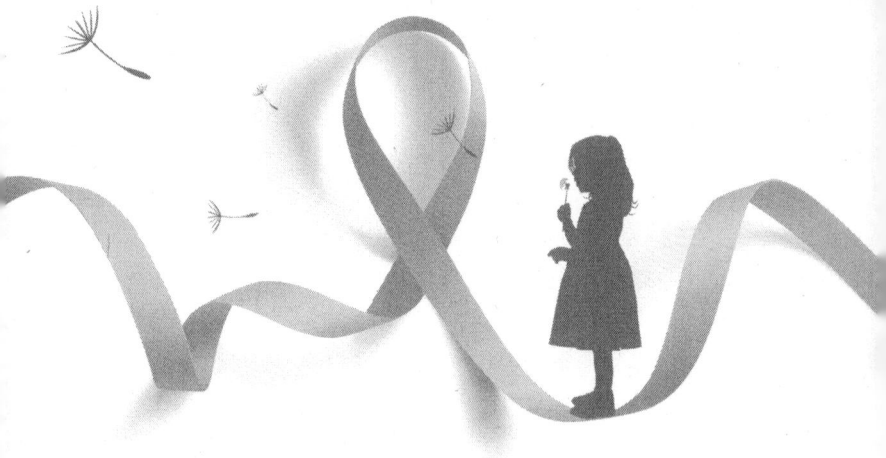

One-way Glass

During the many hours spent sat at Leah's bedside, in and out of the hospital, it is impossible not to think deeply and reflect on life. It sounds really clichéd, but there are so many times when this whole thing has felt like a bad dream. As though I will one day wake up from an incredibly deep sleep and work out that none of this was real – none of it actually happened to us.

I find it so difficult to comprehend that Leah was playing football and running around in the school playground with her friends back in January. Yet, here we are, just seven or eight months later, and things are unrecognisably different. Leah's physical condition during that time has deteriorated rapidly, leaving her struggling to walk, pale-skinned and with threadbare hair. All because of a disease that seems to strike completely at random.

This disease is inordinately cruel. It is indiscriminate.

It sits in the shadows and gradually steals life away from people, often before they even have any opportunity to do anything about it. I hate it. Even the word is painful for me right now. I have been forced to sit and watch as it stole my mother-in-law's life. I have been forced to sit and watch the devastation it has had on Claire, her dad and her sister, as well as the wider family. I have been forced to sit and watch it cause such pain and suffering to my little girl. It has taken her dignity, her strength and some of her sparkle. In the coming few hours, I'm about to find out whether it is going to ultimately take her life. Its final act of cowardice.

From that fateful moment in the ward manager's office at Whiston hospital back in February, when we heard those four words, it felt like we were transported into a parallel universe. To reference *Harry Potter* again, it was like touching a port key and landing in another dimension. An alien world that we know nothing about. A world with a dark, barren landscape. A world where cold winds howl around you day and night and you can never really feel warm or comfortable.

This world, however, has a window. A single large window. The glass in the window is incredibly thick and no matter how hard you bang on it, nobody on the other side can hear you. The window also has one-way glass and nobody on the other side can see you through it. I feel like I'm stood at this window, trying to keep myself warm. Trying to keep Claire and Phoebe and Leah warm, too. We're watching everyone smiling and going about their normal lives through the glass. No one sees or hears us. I feel like we're trapped, and I don't know how to break us out.

Perhaps our only hope of finding our way back to the other side of the glass lies in the hands of these surgeons?

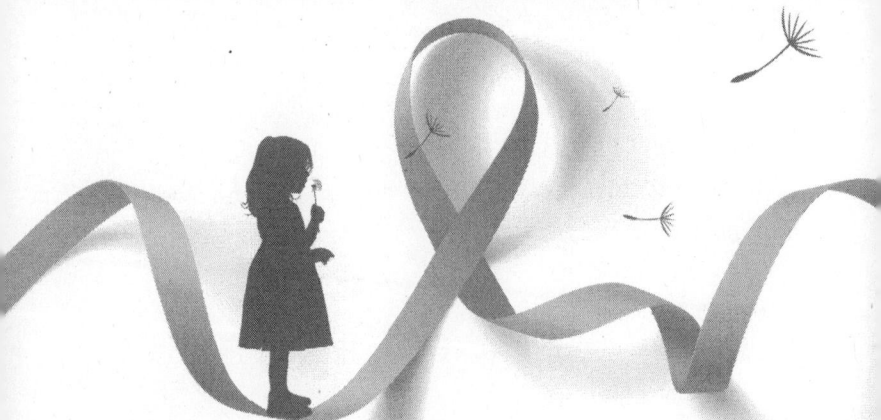

Red Light/Green Light

Thursday 1st August 2019 – 1:37pm

'Hello Harriet, i-i-is everything okay?' I honestly don't know whether I want her to answer that question. I can feel Claire's eyes boring into the side of my head. She knows this is *the* call. I can hear my heart beating hard in my chest.

Harriet proceeds to inform me that her part of the procedure is now complete. More importantly, she tells me it has gone smoothly. She then continues to tell me that she has been asked by the other surgeons to contact us and let us know where things are up to inside the theatre. I close my eyes and inhale deeply.

'The team have reviewed the situation and they have made the decision to try and proceed with the surgery,' says Harriet assertively.

I exhale. 'Oh, thank God for that!' I say.

Claire is still staring at me, trying to gauge what is being said, but her facial expression suggests that she senses it is positive. I flash her a smile, a nod and a thumbs up, and she nods in acknowledgement and punches the air in celebration. I thank Harriet for letting us know and she tells us that the surgical team will try to update us again later. Then, she wishes us all well and ends the call.

The relief to hear that news is indescribable. They are going to give it a shot! She is going to be given the only thing we'd ever asked for since we touched the port key in early February… a chance of survival.

The fact that they are going to attempt to remove this tumour is just everything we have longed to hear. Even so, our relief and excitement is also tinged with a large degree of anxiety. The attempted removal of the tumour was always going to be the hugely risky part of the procedure. Yes, they are going to give her a chance to live, but at the same time they are also now creating the chance that she could die today. My stomach turns over at this thought. I just need to keep hoping the Big Guy Upstairs has read my note on that metal tree.

Thursday 1st August 2019 – 3:30pm

My watch ticks past 3:30pm. We've had no further updates from the theatre since I spoke to Harriet earlier. We are desperate to know how things are going, but even more desperate to know she is still here and she is okay. Claire and I have done another few laps of the park over the last hour. I've managed to eat one full biscuit and Claire managed a bite of one. It's safe to say we both have zero appetite.

My phone has now started to ping with WhatsApp messages from family and close friends…

Any news?
How is she doing?
Thinking of you all xx

I've already relayed the message about the operation proceeding as hoped. I don't have any more news to give them. This is torture for everyone.

A few minutes later, my phone rings – No Caller ID. I swallow deeply. Surely they haven't finished already. If they have… oh God… it might be bad news. I desperately want to answer the call, but I also don't. I take a deep breath.

'H-Hello?' I stutter nervously. It's one of the nurses from ward 3A. She is calling to let us know that there is a room allocated for Leah up there and it is now free. She tells us that we are welcome to go up whenever we are ready. I thank her and end the call. I bow my head and my hand falls away from my ear and back to my side. Phew! No news is definitely good news in some situations.

Claire and I decide that it is probably a good idea to go up to the surgical ward and wait up there in private. It might mean we don't wear the soles of our shoes out or churn up the path round the park, too.

Thursday 1st August 2019 – 5pm

Leah has been in theatre for almost seven hours now. That is a strange thought for me. Surely it cannot be good for her to be under anaesthetic for that long? It does, however, demonstrate the enormity and complexity of the procedure that the team have attempted. It is distressing to think that she's had to go through that, and I still wish every second that I could face it all instead of her. We also know from the conversations we've had with the surgical team that this was never going to be a straightforward, quick procedure. In fact, we were told explicitly that it could take many hours. In my head, the longer she is in the theatre, the more work they are doing and therefore the better chances of success, right?

Regardless of whether or not that is accurate, I have no choice but to keep convincing myself it is true, because the waiting to hear news is excruciating.

Fifteen minutes later, our wait is over.

Thursday 1st August 2019 – 5:15pm

My phone rings. It isn't in my pocket now. It's already in my hand, as I've been staring at it while sat in this room for the last hour. I answer it.

'Hello?'

'Hello, Stephen, it's Jo Minford.'

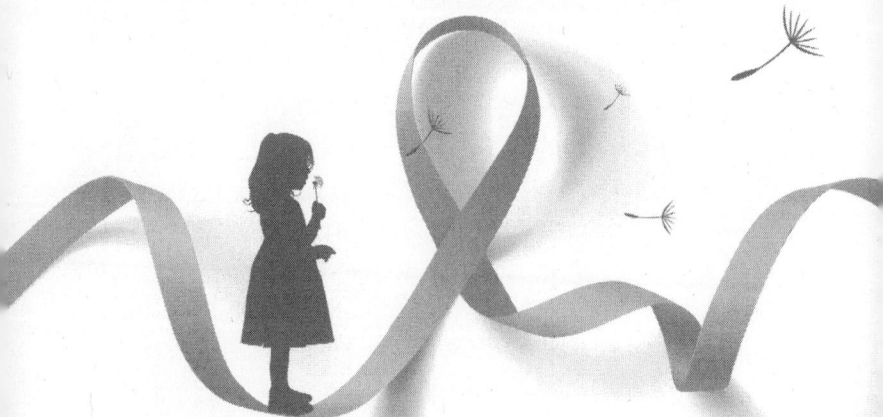

We Could Be Heroes

Thursday 1st August 2019 – 5:16pm

'Hi, Jo. How is she? How is she? Please tell me she's okay, Jo. Is she okay?'

I can feel Claire staring at me again, so I take the phone away from my ear and fumble with it to put it on speakerphone.

'Hi, Stephen. Yes, she's okay. The team are just finishing up now. Can we come up and see you?'

'Yes, of course,' I say. 'We're on 3A.'

'Okay, we'll see you shortly,' says Jo and ends the call.

'What does that mean?' shouts Claire. 'Why are they coming straight up to talk to us? She said she was okay, though, didn't she? She definitely said that, didn't she? Didn't she?'

'Yes,' I reply, 'she definitely said she was okay. She's

okay! Nothing else matters!'

We are both a little shell-shocked and unsure how to interpret the call, but we share a hug and a nervous smile.

Thursday 1st August 2019 – 5:25pm

The door to the room on the ward slides open and Jo Minford and Fiona Murphy walk in. They are both wearing maroon theatre scrubs. Claire and I are standing in the corner of the room, staring at them, eyes wide, hearts racing. Jo breaks the silence straight away.

'So… the *thing* is currently in a bucket and on its way to pathology to be tested. We managed to get it out,' she says.

'And she's okay?' Claire asks.

'Yes, she seems fine. The team are just finishing off now,' Jo replies with a smile on her face.

'*Oh my God, Jo! Thank you! Thank you so much! Thank you for everything! Thank you, Fiona!*'

I have never felt euphoria like it. It was like every demon that had taken over my body over the last few months, fuelled by negative news and difficult situations, had been instantly exorcised. Jo delivered the message as cool as can be, like she does these things every day. I can see she is trying to remain totally professional, but her smile tells me that this is a big deal for her, too.

Claire and I are in floods of tears. I fling my arms around Fiona, who is unfortunate enough to be stood next to me, and give her a huge hug. Claire pounces on Jo at the same time. I'm not sure Jo has ever had a hug like it in her life. Her eyes bulge out of her head slightly as Claire squeezes her tightly. The release of emotion, adrenaline, relief and happiness is completely overwhelming.

They had done it! She had done it! We had all done it! Against all the odds and against the advice of all the other so-called experts. Somehow, *somehow*, they've been proven wrong. Right here, right now is quite simply the most incredible moment of my life. I step back from Fiona and go over to hug Jo, while Claire does the same with Fiona. I notice that both of them are now in tears, too. That professional front can only last so long. It is an unbelievably emotional moment for us all. Really special.

I've dreamt about hearing those words for months and months, and to finally hear them is even better than I could ever have imagined. I immediately think back to that evening in early May when I was sat on the floor in the shower, crying my heart out, with the water running down my face. At that point, I had almost lost hope. I felt like I had hit the bottom. I simply couldn't see this future unfolding. Well, here we are, almost three months later. I think this hospital has saved more than Leah's life today; I think they've possibly saved mine, too.

Claire and I calm down for a second, long enough for Jo and Fiona to describe the next steps. They inform us that Leah is going to be taken to intensive care to be monitored overnight as a precaution. We will get a call to let us know when she is there and when we can go to see her. They then leave the room and leave Claire and I to gather ourselves together. In my mind, I like to think they high five each other outside the room and then skip down the corridor together, but I'm sure that's probably not professional.

Thursday 1st August 2019 – 5:45pm

We know there are a lot of anxious people awaiting news back at home, so we are now desperate to call them and break the news. Claire picks up her phone and calls her dad. He answers straight away.

'Hi, Claire, any news? How is she?'

'They did it, Dad! They did it! They got it out and she's okay. Mum did it for her, Dad! Mum did it for us!'

I hear Claire's voice crack at this point and I hear Peter on the other end of the call sounding emotional, too. It is a beautiful moment that fills my heart. I'm still sobbing softly from twenty minutes earlier, so this conversation just makes the tears flow slightly more.

Claire is going to call Amy next, so I walk over to the other side of the room next to the window and call my mum and dad. It dawns on me that the last time I called them from a hospital window with big news like this, I was telling them that their granddaughter had cancer and turning their world upside down. It feels a little like redemption that I now get to make the call I'm about to make. I press call and my mum picks up the phone within a heartbeat. As soon as she answers, I can hear the tension in her voice.

'Hello, love, is she okay?'

I feel myself getting so choked up, I can barely speak to reply. 'They did it, Mum. She's okay.' I somehow manage to spit some words out.

'Oh God, Ste…' and she moves away from the phone. I know she is in pieces. I can hear her crying. It reminds me a little of the phone call I made to her outside the maternity ward after Phoebe was born and I had just told her that she was a nana.

Phoebe has been with my mum and dad all day and she gets on the phone next. 'Daddy, what's up? Nana is crying. Is Leah not okay?' She sounds terrified.

'No, darling, Leah is fine. Nana is just happy. Those are happy tears.'

'So she's okay? Are you sure?'

'Yes, I'm sure. Mum and I are going to go and see her shortly and we'll tell her you are all thinking about her.'

'Okay, thanks Dad. Love you.'

'Love you, too. Tell Nana I'll call her again later.'

Shortly after, we fire out a quick flurry of text and WhatsApp messages so that our close friends also have the news. Around ten minutes later, my phone rings again. It is one of the lead nurses from the intensive care ward. She tells us that Leah has arrived with them and that she is currently asleep, but is fine. She informs us that we can make our way over to see her as soon as the shift handover is complete at around 7:30pm.

Thursday 1st August 2019 – 7:35pm

When we arrive at intensive care, we are directed to the very end bay of beds. It is a really long ward and it feels like we've had to walk about two miles to get to her. We ask one of the nurses where Leah is. She points to a bed in the far corner. As we approach, I can see her little pale face with her thin wispy hair. She has tubes coming from all corners of her body and the stain of orange iodine across her abdomen. She looks so weak and fragile. In that moment, I decide to take a photo of her as she sleeps. Claire looks at me incredulously, as if to say, 'Why the hell would you want to remember her looking like this?' In truth, this is one of the most important photos I think I've ever taken. I want to be able to show her what she's been through. I want her to understand just how far she has come on her journey. I want her to never forget how proud we are of her.

We chat to the nurse who is looking after her today and she explains all the tubes and various medications that she is hooked up to. It is mainly pain management medication and antibiotics. One of the tubes has the word fentanyl written on it. This is serious pain management.

Around twenty minutes later, Leah rouses slightly and opens her eyes. She is groggy and looks really tired, but she manages to sit up in the bed with the assistance of the nurse.

'Hello, sweetheart,' says Claire. 'You did it, baby! You did it! Me and Daddy are so proud of you.'

I kiss her very gently on the forehead and she musters a smile. It is then that she realises that she has an NG[37] tube coming out of her nose and immediately starts to pull it out. The nurse stops her, but soon agrees that she can probably manage okay without it and so removes it from her, much to Leah's satisfaction. It makes me smile that her

---

37 Nasogastric tube.

first action after waking up following major surgery is to try and pull an unwanted tube from her nose. She's never been frightened to let people know what she wants!

Seeing her sitting up and able to smile after the ordeal that she has been through today is really reassuring and removes some of my anxiety. Now that I've seen her, I know she is okay. I know it is true that she survived the operation. I know she's been given a chance and I know she will take it. I also know how incredibly humble I feel about what has happened to us today. Despite my little girl being sat in a bed in intensive care, with a vast array of tubes covering her body, I feel a strange sense of peace and calm.

'I love you,' I whisper to her.

'I love you plus one,' she whispers back.

Thursday 1st August 2019 – 9pm

Claire and I stay with Leah for just over an hour, but she sleeps for most of that time. There are no beds for parents in intensive care, so we are unable to sleep next to her. The team have kindly spoken to Ronald McDonald House[38] on the edge of the hospital site and arranged a room for us in there for the evening so that we are not too far away. We gratefully accept the room and, after speaking to Leah's

---

38 Ronald McDonald House is a building run by the charity of the same name. Every time you put your change from your Happy Meal into the red collection tins in a McDonald's restaurant, it goes towards these facilities, which allow families to stay close to their children when one of them requires an extended hospital stay.

nurse, we decide it is best to leave her to rest and try and get some rest ourselves.

En route to Ronald McDonald House, we realise that we have barely eaten a thing all day, so we pop across the road to a local fish and chip shop and take our dinner back to the room. It is, without question, one of the best fish and chips I've ever tasted in my life. In truth, it could have been dog food and I'm sure it would have tasted delicious tonight.

At around 10:30pm, the events of the day start to catch up with us and we start to feel fatigued. We both get ready for bed and turn out the lights, but I just lie there in the dark, staring at the ceiling. I still cannot quite believe that we have made it here. I'm shaking my head in disbelief and smiling. I ask myself how the hell do I even begin to thank people for what they've done to help us? How do you possibly repay someone who put their career and reputation on the line to save your child? How can I possibly thank every person who has played a part in this journey? There are so many, after all[39].

Today has simultaneously been the worst and best day of my life. Believe me, that's quite some twenty-four hours! I think it must have been after 2am before the adrenalin subsided enough to allow me to sleep.

---

39 I eventually decided to shine a light on it by writing a book! I'll get round to finishing it one day…

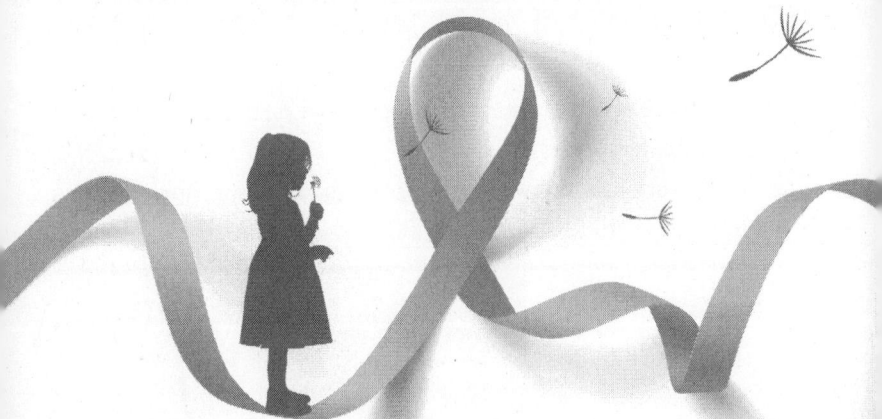

I Got a Feeling

Friday 2nd August 2019

We woke up really early this morning, still buzzing from yesterday's events and the miraculous outcome. We are both still in a bit of a state of disbelief, but absolutely cannot wait to get back across to the hospital to go and see Leah.

At just after 7:30am, we dash back across the car park and go straight back to intensive care. When we arrive, Leah is sat up in bed. She still looks tired and she still has wires and tubes going in and out of her body, but considering what has happened to her, she looks really good.

'Hello, sweetheart, how are you feeling?' I ask immediately and kiss her forehead.

'I'm tired, Daddy… and I'm hungry. Can I have some Rice Krispies?'

I glance over to the nurse, who shakes her head.

'Sorry, but she's not allowed any solid food until her bowel shows signs of getting back to normal. Doctor's orders!' responds the nurse.

It's not the answer she wanted, but it's probably the answer I expected. The fact that she has even asked for some food is amazing. I don't think she has asked for breakfast for at least four months.

I call home a little later in the morning to speak to Phoebe. She is fine and she asks whether she can come in and see Leah. I tell her she can, but only when Leah is back on one of the main wards. Visiting is restricted in intensive care, for obvious reasons. I also speak to my mum and dad, who are still on cloud nine and spent all evening yesterday phoning round the extended family. Today feels like the calm after the storm.

At around 2pm, the nursing team tell us that Leah is well enough to go back to ward 3A and the surgical team have agreed for her to go. Within an hour, the hospital porters arrive to transfer her. She will continue her post-op recovery on 3A for at least another week, but probably two.

I agree to stay in the hospital overnight tonight so that Claire can go back home and see Phoebe. In the early evening, Claire kisses us both and sets off home, leaving Leah and I to settle in for the night.

Leah is sleeping on and off, so I decide to dim the lights in the room so as not to disturb her. Just before 7pm, the door to the room slides open. I look up and in walks Jo Minford. I jump up to greet her.

'Hello, Jo. This is a nice surprise.'

'Hello, Stephen,' she replies. 'I'm off on leave tomorrow, so I just wanted to pop in and check on Leah on my way home.'

Jo then proceeds to check Leah over, paying particular attention to her legs. I assume she is checking that her blood flow to her lower limbs appears normal. All the while, Jo is trying her best not to wake her up.

'She looks great,' Jo says to me.

'She really does, considering what she's been through,' I reply. 'All thanks to you guys, Jo. We can't thank you enough.'

'Well, you did say to us that if we gave her a chance, she would take it!'

I smile at her.

Jo stays in Leah's room chatting to me for over thirty minutes. During that time, she tells me that she herself has been treated for breast cancer recently. She is currently in remission and awaiting the formal 'all-clear'. She tells me that her own experiences have made her appreciate the emotional impact of a cancer diagnosis a little more. After going through treatment herself, she is now determined to do everything in her gift to strike back at this disease. I didn't think I could possibly have more admiration for her than I did after everything she has done for Leah. It turns out, I was wrong!

We go on to chat about our initial meeting and how we both felt about it. Jo tells me that when she realised she knew me, it made the whole conversation even more difficult for her. I've never really thought about whether I felt that conversation was made more difficult because

I knew her beforehand. I think I probably took some comfort in that actually. I certainly didn't feel like I was walking completely into the unknown. Perhaps it also made a tiny difference in terms of her being ever so slightly more invested in Leah's situation? Who knows?

We chat about the incredible 3D model that she made and how much that changed things for us all. Jo tells me that having the ability to see and touch the tumour in 3D form made a huge difference to her and the surgical team, too. It allowed them to plan the approach to surgery more thoroughly and helped them to communicate the plan to all relevant people involved before the 'live show'. I suspect it might just have been the reason Jo and the team felt confident to try the surgery. Again, who knows? What I do know, though, is that it turns out that this is the first time a 3D model has been used successfully to attempt this type of cancer surgery in the UK. My mind is blown again.

Just before she leaves, Jo tells me one final thing. She says that she doesn't really know why she made the decision to take the procedure on. 'I just had a feeling. I had a feeling that maybe we could do this. Maybe we could just find a way to make this work. I can't explain it, but I just had a feeling.'

Claire is utterly convinced that 'feeling' has a lot to do with her mum. I'm struggling to find a way to disagree. After all, there's always a way, right?

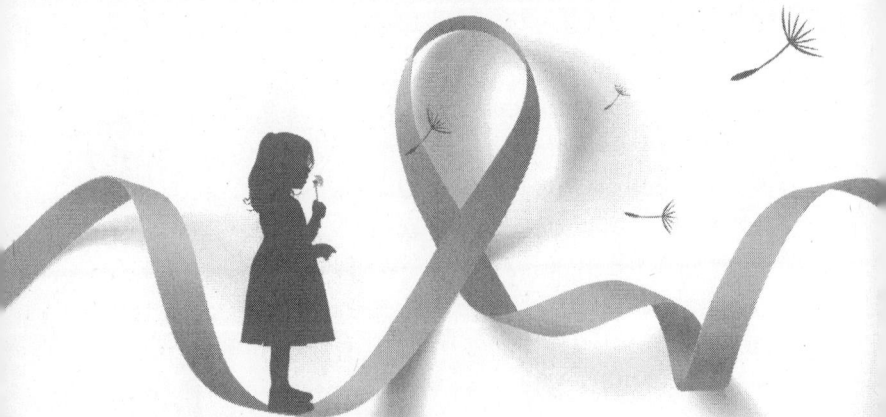

Our Happy Place

Over the course of the next two weeks, Leah steadily recovers from the operation. All of the other surgeons who operated on her come back in to check on her progress in the days following the procedure. All of them are pleased with how the operation has gone and all are pleased with Leah's progress. Seeing them all individually gives us another opportunity to thank them personally. Each time, it is an emotional moment. These people are total heroes!

Gradually, Leah starts to get back on her feet and walk small distances around the ward, as well as starting to eat small amounts of food again. On the 14th of August, Leah is deemed well enough to go home. Just a week before her seventh birthday.

We manage to get a short break up to the house in Scotland for a few days over her birthday week. It is the first occasion we have spent any time as a family away from the house or Alder Hey all year. Leah turning seven feels like an enormous milestone. There were many moments during the darkest times when I questioned whether she would make it to her seventh birthday. Instead, she spent it riding round a park on an island off the west coast of Scotland on a kid's quad bike. If someone had told me that back in May, I'm not sure even the greatest optimist within me could have believed it. I actually feel somewhat guilty for allowing myself to doubt this outcome was possible now. Perhaps that is the difference that Claire's faith made to her, and to us all?

Returning to the house in Scotland is bittersweet for us all. It felt beautiful to be there with Leah, watching her smile and seeing 'the old Leah' gradually returning. However, it is also tinged with sadness that Marie is not able to be here with us. The house is full of decorative touches that instantly make you think of her. In some ways, even though she isn't here with us, at the same time she was everywhere, all around us.

In September 2019, Leah's care is handed over to the Clatterbridge Cancer Centre under Dr Thorp, as planned. Her next course of treatment requires us to take her across to the Wirral every Monday to Friday morning for six and a half weeks. In total, she receives thirty-three doses of high-grade radiotherapy. The treatment is aimed at her general abdominal area with specific concentration on the areas of known residual disease[40]. The care Leah receives at Clatterbridge is faultless and the transition of her care

---

40 I.e. the small sections of tumour that were unable to be removed by surgery.

across to another organisation is seamless. Dr Thorp, as a member of the MDT at Alder Hey, knew Leah's condition and our family's situation in depth and it really doesn't feel at all like she is receiving care in another hospital.

During this time, Leah also starts to return to school gradually. Just the odd afternoon at first when she was feeling up to it, but building up slowly. She ends up having to go back into Alder Hey on a handful of occasions across September and October due to abdominal pain and bowel discomfort. These turn out to be fairly standard side effects of the radiotherapy treatment, but, generally, she tolerates the treatment well considering the intensity of the dose.

In late September, she got the opportunity to attend her very first Premier League football match when she is kindly given complimentary tickets to the Everton vs Manchester City game at Goodison Park, courtesy of Everton Football Club. After the match, she is invited into the tunnel to meet some of the players and get autographs. She loves the experience and shouts her heart out for the whole game. The irony is not lost on me that this was the fixture she missed back in February 2019, the day before her initial diagnosis. It makes it all the more special, though. I just wish Everton bothered to turn up, too!

In mid-October, Leah receives her final dose of radiotherapy, and a few weeks later, Prof. Pilling informs us of the decision not to bring Leah back in for any further treatment. The hope now is that the surgery and subsequent radiotherapy have done enough to prevent further growth/spread of the tumour. We hope so, too, and we are thrilled to hear that she doesn't need any further chemo treatment.

Throughout November, Leah starts to return to school full-time and manages to complete her first full week back in school in early December. In mid-December, she is back to theatre for the fifth time to have her broviac line removed. This means she can start to go swimming again. Each small achievement is another huge step towards normality for her and us all. She remains fit and well throughout the rest of December and we enjoy spending Christmas and New Year together as a family.

Her next MRI scan is on Friday 3rd January 2020 and we discuss the results with Barry the following week. Everything looks okay and the residual disease visible in her abdominal muscle has actually reduced in size. Barry puts Leah onto three-monthly monitoring from that moment onwards and she won't need to come into the hospital between scans unless we have any concerns. She goes back to theatre for the sixth time on Tuesday 21st January to finally have her gastrostomy tube removed.

In early January, both Claire and I return to work after eleven months off. It feels strange going back after such a long time. Adapting back to 'normal' life after such a turbulent and traumatic year takes quite a lot of adjustment.

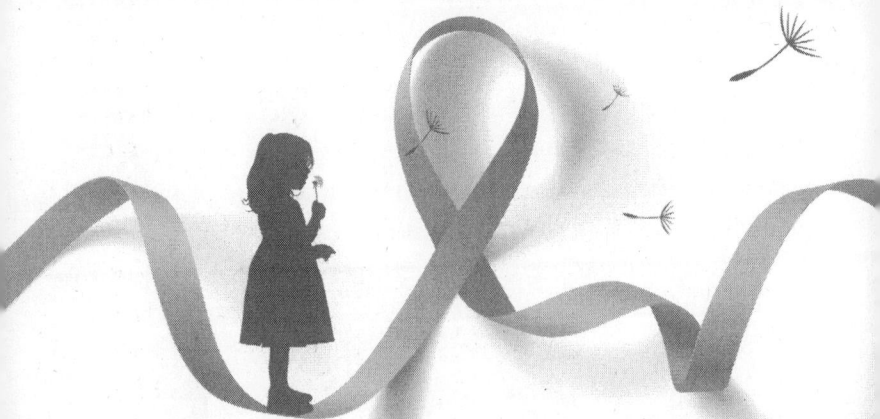

Ring It Loud and Proud

On Monday 27th January 2020, almost exactly one year after that fateful visit to the GP, Leah finally gets her moment as she stands in front of her family and the staff on Ward 3B and rings the end-of-treatment bell at Alder Hey. It is, without doubt, the proudest moment of our lives.

I don't want to miss the opportunity to give personal thanks to the incredible staff at the hospital who cared for her (and us) over the last twelve months and ultimately saved her life (and ours). Therefore, I read out a speech I had written to let them know what we thought of them.

I just wanted a minute of your time to say a few words about the journey that we, as a family, have been on for the last twelve months and how you have all helped play a role in how we have ended up stood here today.

February 6th 2019 – a date I will unfortunately never, ever forget. The day, my near-perfect world completely fell apart after hearing just four simple words... your child has cancer. Words that no parent should ever have to hear. Almost twelve months later, having been on the toughest journey of our lives, we've finally made it to the point where we get to stand beside our daughter and celebrate what this brave and inspirational little girl has achieved in getting the better of this evil, cowardly disease.

But the truth is, no matter how much courage and determination Leah has shown, she could not have achieved this on her own. Without the army of carers, helpers and supporters who have graced our lives along the way, it's probably not untrue to say that she wouldn't be here with us now to enjoy this moment.

Many of you will have heard the widely used anecdote about when US president John F Kennedy visited NASA HQ in 1961 and introduced himself to a janitor who was mopping the floor. When he asked the janitor what he did at NASA, the Janitor replied, 'Me, Sir? I help put men on the moon.'

Well, I think the exact same principle behind that statement also holds true in Leah's case and in the case of the many hundreds of children that you look after here in the oncology service at Alder Hey. Each and every one of you plays a crucial role in helping these children and their families navigate through the unthinkable by making the journey a tiny bit more bearable at every opportunity.

From the immensely talented surgeons and their anaesthetists and theatre teams, who ignored all those up and down the country who said Leah's tumour was

*'inoperable' and that surgery 'wasn't in her best interests',
and showed bravery and skill on a level I never knew existed
to remove it. To the amazing play specialists on the ward
who have always been on hand with strategic Play-Doh and
a hug whenever Leah's felt down.*

*From the wonderful cleaners, who not only keep this
place spotless and safe, but also take the time to chat and
make Leah feel at home whenever she has to spend time
on the ward. To the brilliant oncology medical team and
particularly Prof Pilling (or should we say Princess Pilling),
who have worked relentlessly and pushed hard to get the best
possible outcome for Leah from day one, whatever it took.*

*From the incredible team of nurses on the ward who
have put up with Leah's whoopee cushions, plastic snakes
and horrible flavoured jelly beans, and have always been on
hand with a sick bowl, a smile and sometimes just a warm
word of encouragement when it is needed. To the excellent
chefs in the kitchen who have served up whatever Leah has
wanted whenever she has wanted it and helped keep her
strength up (always with a Freddo on the side).*

*From the fantastic housekeeper and healthcare
assistants, who make the best toast in the world after nights
of broken sleep and sky-high anxiety. They also never failed
to get Leah's TV working to help her through a six-night stay
in hospital. To the absolutely fabulous community outreach
team, who have been alongside us throughout, as a shoulder
to cry on or to provide a word of encouragement when
desperately needed.*

*Not to mention Mike (Nugget), Eddie and the other
charities that have helped us through, Jo in the classroom,*

the pharmacy team, the OTs, dieticians, physios, radiology team and probably hundreds of others that I've missed. This has been a true team effort and you should all be proud of the individual parts you have each played in getting us here.

You may not help put men on the moon like the janitor at NASA, but you all contribute to something even more incredible… you help to save children's lives.

When I worked here a few years ago, there was a marketing campaign being run by the charity called 'the land of remarkable people' and today that strapline has never felt more appropriate. This is an impressive hospital, there is no doubt about that, but what makes it truly remarkable is the people who work in it… all of you. You are not just doctors, nurses, pharmacists, teachers, cleaners or 'admin', you have become friends and almost part of our family.

Each and every one of you has gone above and beyond to make this horrible journey slightly more bearable and to keep us believing that we could somehow get Leah to the end. You have never given up on our daughter and you have taught us that miracles can happen.

God bless you all and, from the bottom of our hearts, thank you.

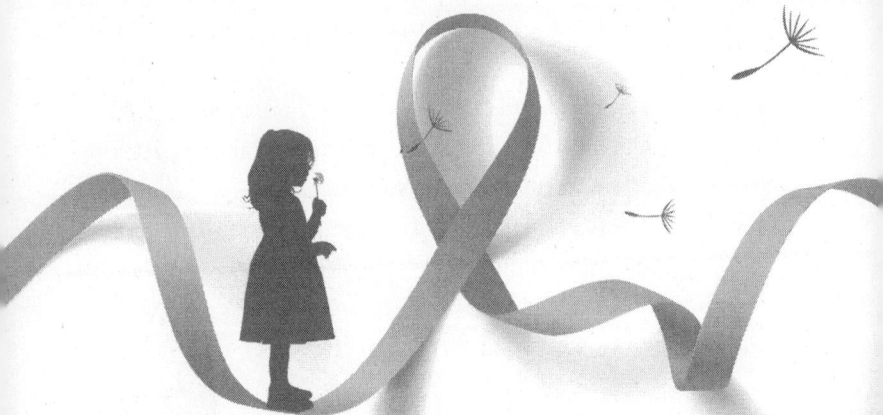

Yesterday, Tomorrow, Today

Since ringing the bell in January 2020, life for Leah, and all of us, has been a bit of a roller coaster. After much deliberation, Claire and I decided to share the story in the local press. It then quickly ended up in the *Daily Mail* and, a few days later, Leah appeared on the BBC Breakfast's famous red sofas, alongside myself and Jo Minford, to talk about her experience[41].

Less than two months later – ahead of a summer that we had packed full of fun once-in-a-lifetime adventures – the whole world changed again. This time, though, it changed for everyone else, too, as the Covid-19 pandemic struck. It wiped out every single one of our plans and

---

41 Over a million people have subsequently watched Leah's interview on Facebook.

hugely increased anxiety as Leah was now in the 'at risk' category. However, when life has dealt you all some pretty poor hands in the past, living through a global pandemic, for us, felt strangely insignificant. Despite the trauma and devastation experienced by many people around us, we were quite content to exist in our little bubble.

In late 2020, as the latest national lockdown eased off, Leah achieved yet another thing that I had more or less given up hope of happening. She pulled on her football boots and stepped back onto the pitch to play football with her old team. It was another momentous milestone on her journey and another opportunity for me to have a little cry.

Despite the challenges of the pandemic, 2020 was a year where our family stepped further and further away from the darkness that had engulfed us the year before. Sadly, as we had now become painfully accustomed to, the roller coaster of life brings downs as well as ups.

In early December that year, following a routine MRI scan, Barry informed us that he had some concerns over the results. There was evidence of new growth within the areas of residual disease in and around Leah's spine. Immediately, the positivity that we had been cautiously building was replaced by a familiar sense of fear and uncertainty. Christmas 2020 was extremely difficult, trying to enjoy ourselves and have fun with the girls, while simultaneously being terrified about the situation that we potentially found ourselves in once more.

Leah's scan was repeated in early January and, soon after, it was confirmed that she had indeed relapsed. Our hearts, which we had been steadily supergluing back together over recent times, were broken once again.

We knew that she hadn't really responded well to the original chemo treatment back in 2019, so it was highly unlikely that further inpatient chemo would be an option. We started to discuss surgical options with Barry. Due to the location of the residual disease and the fact that she had subsequently undergone radiotherapy treatment, surgery was again deemed to be extremely high risk and was therefore not really a good option. Things were not looking great again for us.

However, there was some positive news. Back in 2019, we had consented for samples of the tumour removed from Leah's abdomen to be sent off for genetic testing. The results from some of the tests carried out had been positive. They suggested that the tumour contained a known gene mutation found in rare cancers and this meant that there was potentially a treatment available to Leah that hadn't previously been considered.

Subsequently, she commenced the drug treatment in January 2021. The drug is taken at home twice a day and, to date, Leah has managed the treatment exceptionally well. Her scans since that date have shown no further progression from the residual disease, which is brilliant news. She continues to attend school full-time and continues to enjoy life playing football and playing out with her friends. She is quite simply incredible – and long may she continue to be incredible!

The picture below was taken in March 2022 as she celebrated her Holy Communion with her friends from school[42]. This is three years after that fateful day when she was diagnosed.

Take a look…

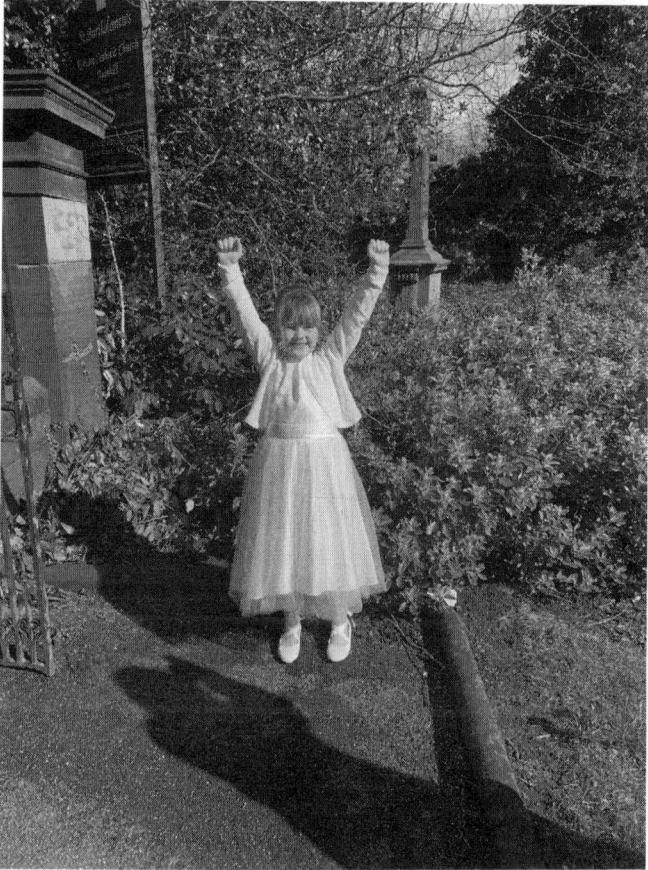

… and then tell me that the decision to remove that tumour was 'not in her best interests'.

---

42 *Another* huge milestone she has passed.

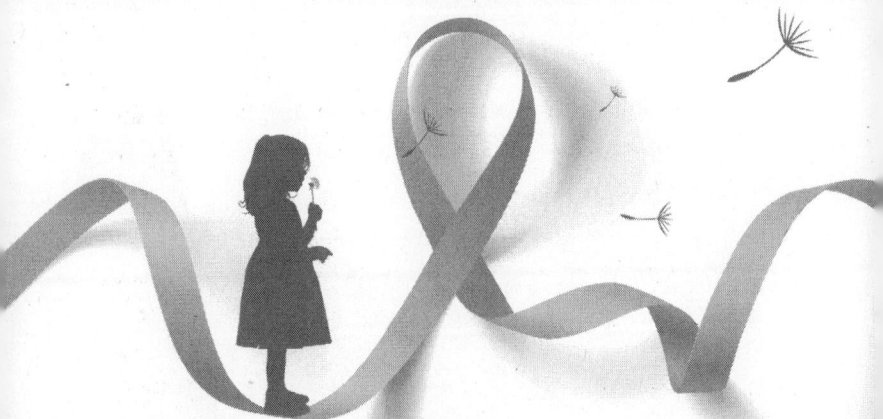

Epilogue

When your child is diagnosed with a serious illness, it devastates you, them and everyone around you. It creates a level of anxiety that never truly leaves you; you just have to learn to manage it over time. You continually have to hold out hope that the day-to-day anxiety never becomes grief of loss.

The children diagnosed with cancer, on the other hand, especially younger children, seem to generally deal with everything in their stride and approach everything with incredible determination that you would not expect to find in someone of such a young age. Leah always tries hard to see the fun side of life and always wears a smile no matter what is thrown her way. She's really inspirational for us all and for other people I know who have dealt with personal difficulties (including cancer battles). They have told me that Leah has inspired them through their treatment.

This book is an incredibly personal account of the toughest period of my life. I struggled immensely to continue to be the dad, the husband, the son, the brother and the friend that I knew I had to be. At the same time, just trying to hold myself together and keep standing up every day became huge challenges. In time, as I have learned to reflect and process the events of the past, I have appreciated more and more the importance of hope. Hope is the very fuel that keeps your engine running when times get tough. I found that people either helped to top up your engine or they drained it.

There are many reasons why I chose to put Leah's journey into writing:

I have found that writing about Leah's story and talking about it as often as possible has helped me to mentally process the scale of what happened to her and my family. It has helped me to understand it and learn to accept it.

We are keen to see all those individuals that have helped us along the way get the recognition they truly deserve. The bravery of the Alder Hey surgical team to make the decision to attempt surgery when all other hospitals around the country said no is beyond inspiring, and came with considerable personal and professional risk to each of them. They put their professional reputations on the line to save our little girl and we can't thank them enough. We want them to be held up as heroes for what they did (even though they will probably cringe at the thought!). Also, it is important to note that the surgeons only played one of the roles in Leah's story and, before surgery was possible, Leah received incredible care from the oncology team and a huge number of other teams and individuals inside and outside Alder Hey. I would love each and every one of them to know that they played a part in getting Leah back on her feet and keeping her going through the toughest times. Sometimes even the smallest things that people do to help have the biggest impact; there are lots of examples of tiny things that people have done for us over the last year and they probably do not realise how much of an impact they had on us and our ability to cope with the magnitude of what was happening.

Back in May 2019, when we lost Marie and we were being told that surgery was not looking likely for Leah, we were desperately searching to find hope from any source we could find. We were desperate to speak to or hear from someone whose child had been through Leah's situation and survived. The reality was that there were no examples. Therefore, we had to put all our hope and faith in Leah being the first person to do it. Now that we are here, Claire and/or I can become the people that we needed to speak to/hear from all those months ago. I hope that Leah's story might just be what another family needs to hear to keep them going. Miracles can happen and you should never, ever give up.

We would like to help raise awareness of childhood cancer and the signs and symptoms. It was a simple article on the BBC website that prompted us to take Leah back to the GP for another medical opinion. Perhaps this decision ultimately gave the clinical teams enough time to identify her illness and then subsequently save her life? Wider awareness of the signs of childhood cancers can, and will, save lives. General awareness of childhood cancer and the devastating impact it has on so many lives will also help with fundraising for cancer research charities who potentially hold the key to finding better treatments and eventually cures. Awareness = Funding = Research = Cure.

We would like to highlight and recognise the importance of effective partnership working in complex cases such as Leah's. Over the course of her treatment, Leah experienced seamless transition of care between Alder Hey and Clatterbridge (and back again), the benefits of sharing opinions and advice with other experts (Prof. Bannan's input from Manchester), multidisciplinary operating teams (Prof. John Brennan's vascular expertise during surgery) and the power of national and international collaboration (discussion at the national sarcoma panel and opinions from surgeons at Memorial Sloane Kettering Cancer Center in New York). There is no doubt all of this contributed to the positive outcome for Leah.

We would like to highlight the impact of innovation and medical advancement and the fact that the 3D model of the tumour facilitated greater planning and confidence in the surgical team. We are aware that since Leah's operation, the approach used on Leah has subsequently been used on other children to give them a chance at life, too. It is really nice to know that all the heartache and pain that Leah and our family went through during 2019 was not in vain and, as a result, not only is Leah still here and thriving, but other children and their families now also have hope where it perhaps never existed.

I hope this book has given you a glimpse into the lives

of those families living 'behind the glass' in the world of childhood cancer. If it helps just one person or family to cope with the challenges for just one more day, then it has served its purpose.

Our family continue to live in a challenging world of uncertainty and we have no idea what the future holds for us. But, undoubtedly, we are the lucky ones. There are so many families we have met along the way who were not so lucky. I send them all my thoughts and my love, always.

Rest in peace, Jaxon, Grace, Lincoln and many, many more.

Far too many.